WHO-DA-THUNKIT

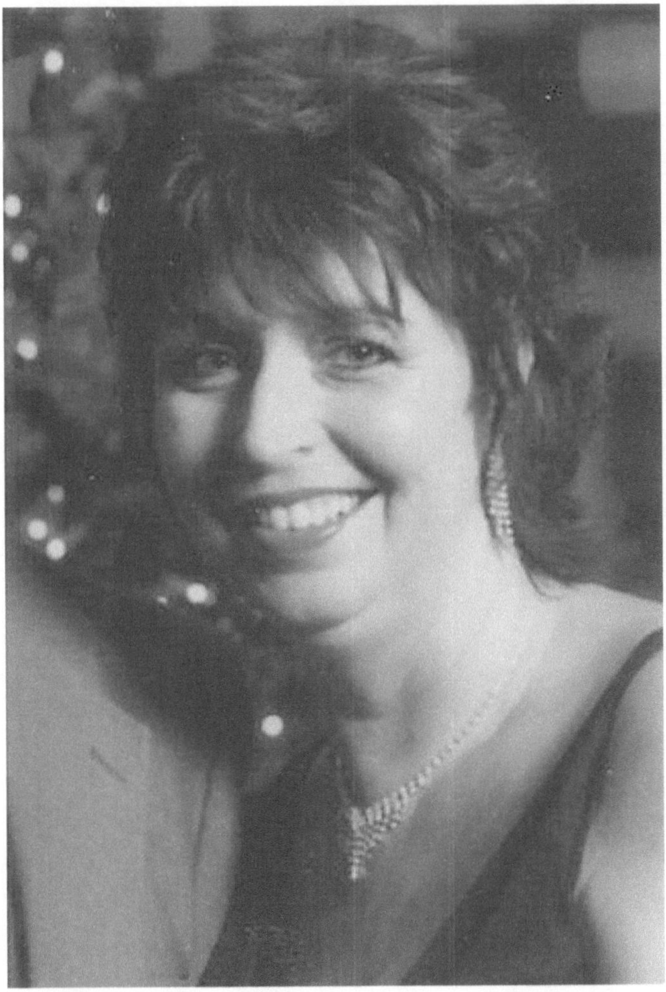

WHO-DA-THUNKIT

Rick Maxwell

Library of Congress Control Number:		2009904912
ISBN:	Hardcover	978-1-4415-3837-6
	Softcover	978-1-4415-3836-9

To order additional copies of this book, contact:
Xlibris Corporation
1-888-795-4274
www.Xlibris.com
Orders@Xlibris.com
62990

CONTENTS

DEDICATION

Dedicated to my wife, Paula Dye Maxwell, whom I love so much.

She has been such an inspiration to me and many others who have come in contact with her. Her faith and strength have been so strong throughout this battle with cancer.

To MD Anderson Cancer Center at the University of Texas who have been instrumental in the care and treatment of my wife.

Also to the pastor, deacons, and congregation of Belmont Baptist Church, Morgantown, Kentucky, who prayed for and anointed Paula.

To everyone who has contributed in any way to make it possible for us to travel to Texas.

And finally, to our family and friends who has been so helpful with cards, letters, and phone calls and prayers in support of her recovery. Without this inspiration, this would have been more difficult than anyone could imagine.

ACKNOWLEDGEMENTS

Paula and I would like to thank the following people and businesses for their support and prayers during this experience.

Donnie and Cathy Sims who helped us with travel plans, and who also stepped into the role of mother as well as sister, since Paula's mother is ill with Alzheimer's disease.

Natasha Widner, Mike and Edwina Cannon who have prayed for us, gave words of encouragement, and helped with the care of the boys while we were away.

Dwayne and Jonell Alford for their moral support and help with food when we were not able to fix our meals.

Teddy Webb for carrying the work load while I was out, and for watching out for our home.

Bruce Maxwell for keeping Paula in his prayers and lighting a candle each day for her.

The pastor, deacons and congregation of Belmont Baptist Church for their prayers. This helped so much.

Bowling Green Municipal Utilities and all of the employees who have supported Paula and held benefits on her behalf.

Employees of the City of Bowling Green Kentucky for their prayers and financial support through the benefits held by BGMU employees.

The entire Dye family for the benefit held in honor of Paula.

Joelyn Yurchison for taking good care of our pets while we were away.

Kimberly Baez and Melanie Barker for their contribution of proceeds from a bake sale.

INTRODUCTION

This is a true story of the daily struggles, tears, and laughter of a cancer patient and caregiver who are newly married. Although there are many options available to any individual with cancer or other catastrophic illness, sometimes you have to put priorities in line and go to the place that can and will offer the best care and treatment no matter the cost. We have laughed, cried, and shouted with joy at good news.

For us it was MD Anderson Cancer Center in Houston, Texas. The travel expenses have been phenomenal, but the experiences on this journey have been joyful, fulfilling, and heartbreaking.

As a caregiver and husband, I have seen the effects of chemotherapy, radiation, and infections that have ravaged my wife's body and soul. I have hurt when she hurts, and I have cried within, and no one knew about it. I have met people from all walks of life with cancer, made new friends, and have a new insight on how precious life can be and how short our lives are.

I hope this will be an inspiration to someone as to how difficult but rewarding life can be with someone you love who has been diagnosed with cancer. There are going to be bad times, but there will be more good times to enjoy with your family. I have learned to never take anything for granted because we really do not know how long we have in this world. Enjoy the weather each day, whatever it may be, watch children play, and walk whenever possible to see everything God has put here for us to see.

THE BEGINNING

September 11, 2001, brought a lot of changes to every community. It was the day that started a whole new life for me as an electrical inspector for a small city in South Central Kentucky.

That fateful day changed the routine I had followed since moving to Bowling Green in June of 1994. I would go do the electrical inspections that had been called in by contractors; at the end of the day or the next morning, I would go to the local utility company and drop them off in the basement to the service department supervisor. But all of that changed and I had to start taking my inspection certificates to the main entrance and log them in there. Not that I am a terrorist, but safety precautions. I followed this routine day in and day out. Until one day, several months later, I noticed a lady, which I had seen working at another job, was working there.

I walked over to the counter and spoke to her, and we struck up a casual conversation, and I noticed another woman there. Paula was her name. She was so cheerful when she spoke to the customers in person or on the phone that she brought a smile to my face. I did not speak to her much at first, but as time went on, we began to talk whenever I would deliver my certificates. After getting to know her, I discovered that she was a woman full of life who keeps a picture of her two boys on her computer monitor for everyone to see.

One day, it was about 10:00 a.m., the sun was shining, the birds were chirping, and the sky was so blue, Paula asked, "What are you going to do now?" And I remarked, "I'm going fishing," which is my passion and has been for some time now. She seemed to light up when I would tell her of my fishing trips and being in the outdoors. A couple of years had passed, and every day I would go in just looking for her, to see her smile and to hear her voice.

January 2006, I felt that there was an attraction between us, so I burned a CD with a couple of songs, and early one morning, I anonymously dropped it off at the side door of her office building in an envelope with her name on it and drove off to do my daily round of inspections. The next day, I received a call from her, asking if I would meet her for lunch, which I was scared to death to do because little did I know that she and a fellow employee had reviewed a surveillance video and found out that it was me.

So we met and talked about the CD and our lives at that time. It seemed as though both of us were in unhappy marriages and lonely for companionship. At the time, she was in the process of a divorce.

Over a period of time, we developed a friendship like I have never known. We began dating, and all was going great. Paula showed me new things and experiences I had not known since I was a young boy. We went to movies and walked in the woods. It was fantastic, almost like being young again. Over the months we did a variety of things.

One day in January, we decided to take off from work early and drive to Nolin Lake where we fished from the bank. It was so cold, and the fish were not biting, but we had a great day being together. While driving to the lake, Paula looked at me and said **"whodathunkit,"** which from then on has been a catchphrase for us. It means who would have thought that the two of us would have gotten together.

February 14, Valentines Day came, and I had a dozen red roses delivered to her workplace. When the delivery man brought them, she had no idea they were for her as she had told me once that "every one gets flowers except me," so that made me feel really good. She was so happy to get those flowers I thought she would never take her eyes off of them. One of her coworkers, Gretta, and she fought over them because Gretta took them and put them on her desk so people would think they were hers. It was funny to see them carry on like that. At that time, Gretta gave me the nickname Romeo because of the things I would do for Paula, such as little notes and other small things. Paula said that it is the little things that mean the most. We did so many things throughout the year; it passed so quickly.

In October of 2006, Paula, her boys, Brad and Logan, and I left Bowling Green on an adventure, going to Myrtle Beach, South Carolina. I had never seen an ocean before and would experience it with her for the first time.

We drove all day into the evening, finally arriving at our destination, checked into the hotel, and walked down to the beach where Paula asked, "What do you think?" I responded, "It looks like a big Kentucky Lake, I'm ready to go home now." To which she got real down about; you could see the disappointment on her face until I told her I was kidding. The next day, we drove to the campground where my oldest brother, Bruce, had a camper trailer parked. Paula, Brad, and Logan finally got to meet Bruce and my other brother, Melvin, who had driven from Madisonville, Tennessee, to visit with us.

AND THE SEASONS CHANGE

Winter came, and we shared Thanksgiving with her family of which I was apprehensive to meet, fearful I would not live up to their expectations. Her family was just great and accepted me with open arms. She comes from a fairly large close-knit family. At holidays, her niece, nephew, sisters, brothers-in-law, and aunt and uncle get together and have dinner. It is really neat since I come from a very small family of four brothers, which I very rarely see. Christmas came and went, and before I knew it, we had been dating for a year. Time sure went fast. January came, and we celebrated our first year of dating. On the weekends that her boys were with their father, we would go to Nashville or some other place and explore stores, little shops, or just have fun doing nothing at all. Sometimes, we would just lie around and watch a movie or go to the lake and walk around.

We got through the cold weather, and spring was just around the corner. We decided to go camping and slept in a tent; even though I had a heater that kept it fairly warm, it can still be cold in March in Kentucky. We walked in the woods, went fishing, and sat around the campfire. To see her in the great outdoors was a joy because she had not experienced this kind of life too much since she was younger when her parents would go camping.

April came, and we were getting ready for spring. By now I had made up my mind that I was going to ask Paula to marry me. I was trying to find the right time and place to do it, but I had so many places in mind. I could ask her at Nolin Lake, which was a special place for us. As it was our first "date," I could take her to a little restaurant we both like; sometimes we would go there for lunch. Or I could ask her at her office. There were just so many places for me to choose from.

OUR NEW LIFE BEGINS

It was Friday evening in April of 2007 when we decided to go to Nashville. We had dinner in a historic restaurant downtown, and I thought about a horse-drawn-carriage ride. What a perfect place to propose marriage to someone you really love. We were riding in the carriage when the driver asked if we were married, and I said, "No, but if she will have me." And I showed her the ring. She looked at me with this look like "what are you doing," and then she realized that I was proposing marriage. I was so afraid that she would say no because we had only been dating for a year, and we still had a lot to learn about one another. Then she squealed "yes, she would marry me," and I was so relieved. We talked a lot about marriage for a while, and that not only would I be marrying her, I would be getting two boys as well. It sure would be a different world, but I was willing to try.

Early on in our relationship, her eldest son, Brad and I had some problems as he did not want to share his mother with someone else because she had done everything with him. We worked through these problems, and he was so excited when she told him that we were getting married that he ran around her house three times. Her youngest son, Logan, did not really grasp the concept, but he was all right with the idea. We continued from then on, making plans and trying to figure out the date and the time of the wedding and most of all the place. We had been to a place at Land Between the Lakes called Patti's Settlement, which is built in the traditional 1800s style. They have a petting zoo for children, a very neat restaurant, and a small chapel. Very small. We had talked about using it because it was such a romantic place. But we decided that it was too small to hold the people we would invite. It would only seat about twelve people.

One Sunday, we drove to a place called Little Bend, a small community in Butler County, where her parents had a farm. And there was small one-room country church where her mother had attended, as a child growing up, and was a member. So I thought this is the perfect place. We both agreed because Paula had thought of the same church. Now we have the place, what about the date? So Saturday, September 22, 2007, was the date we would be married.

This very old church built in 1904 sits back from the road nestled in the trees. It was built with stone pillars, original wood siding, stained glass windows, and the most beautiful interior. But one glitch—no air conditioning, no bathroom. Hopefully, it would be cool on our wedding day. We went one evening for the rehearsal, and everything went pretty well. On the way home, everyone who would take place in the wedding stopped at Farmboy, a restaurant in Morgantown, Kentucky, ate dinner, and discussed the details.

Everything was coming together as we planned our wedding and honeymoon, a cruise to the Bahamas' Islands, something neither of us had done before. We were both so excited; we went shopping for a wedding dress at a couple of places. Paula tried on several dresses to use as decoys so I would not know which one she would get.

A few days later, she and her niece Natasha went back to the bridal shop in Glasgow, Kentucky, and found the perfect dress. She also had the boys fitted for their tuxedos at another shop. They were so handsome. Time was drawing near, and everything was right on schedule.

I called Paula one evening and asked her to wear something light and breezy the next day as I had a plan. I hitched my boat to my truck, called her before lunch and asked her to meet me at a park that is on the Barren River. We met, and I took her by the hand, led her over the hill to which I said to her, "Your chariot awaits." The compact disc player was playing the same song that I had left at the door of her office. She started to cry. She was so pleased with this day; the sky was blue, the birds were singing, and the grass was green.

We took a ride up the river and stopped beside a tree that had fallen into the river, ate sandwiches that I had brought, and just enjoyed the little time we had together.

The times we shared were simple, but so pleasing, and we enjoyed each other's company so much. Time had passed so quickly that it seemed like a whirlwind was taking control.

Finally, the "big day," September 22, arrived, and we were getting married. Everyone we had invited had arrived at the church, and the day was beautiful. Crystal clear skies, warm weather, and all of our friends and family gathered together. As I was standing at the altar, the music started to play and the door opened to reveal an angel standing there—the dress, the accessories, and the tiara shining in the light. I was mesmerized by the beauty of the woman coming down the aisle to take my hand in holy matrimony.

I could not take my eyes off of her; she was so beautiful to me that I barely heard what Brother Gary Embry was saying to me. We exchanged our vows, and during the lighting of our unity candle, we had the same song play that had started our relationship.

Afterward, we left the church headed for Beaver Dam, Kentucky, to a hotel conference room that had been reserved for our reception, where most of our friends shared our joy with the traditional cake and punch. We opened our gifts, took lots of photos, laughed, and got ready to leave Beaver Dam, headed for Fort Lauderdale, Florida, then from there to the Bahamas. We drove late into the night so that we would not have to drive through Atlanta the next morning. We stopped in Forsythe, Georgia, and stayed the night, went to a local steak house, where we sat on opposite sides of the table, held hands, and looked goggle-eyed at each other. Early the next morning, we left for Florida, which was a short trip to me. We arrived at Port Everglades, parked the car, and made our way with luggage in tow to the ship. It was not a large ship, but we were so excited it appeared to be a mile long. Paula squealed with joy, "We're going on a cruise." And we boarded the *Regal Empress,* got our photograph made in front of a backdrop of a life preserver. We made our way down a hallway of dark mahogany wood, to our stateroom, which was small. But who needs a lot of room when you are on a cruise ship, especially when you are on your honeymoon?

Paula had been concerned because she had never been on a cruise, and it was September, hurricane season. I had never been on a cruise either, but I was too excited to think about any of that. The ship departed the port, and we were on our way to a new adventure of visiting paradise for the first time. We stood on deck and watched as the port slowly got farther away, and we enjoyed some fruity drinks and sailed into the vast ocean. We walked around, getting familiar with the ship and taking in all of the sights around us.

Dinner was served around 6:00 p.m., and after dinner we went outside to enjoy the warm air and the smell of the ocean water. We were in love, and it was a beautiful night. We stayed up late that first evening; neither one of us could sleep. The next morning, I had planned for us to go on deck and enjoy the sunrise to which Paula was very receptive. We got up and went topside, excited about seeing a sunrise over the ocean, only to see a pouring-down rain when we walked through the door. We were so bummed that we would not see the sunrise. We went back to the stateroom and went back to sleep. The hum of the engines and the gentle motion of the ship sailing on the ocean made it possible to sleep well.

When we woke up the second time and got showered, we went to breakfast and were to report to the entertainment area for stage shows, and pick up our passes for the beach excursion, which we had previously paid. We were disappointed to find out that the excursion had been cancelled due to the weather, so we chose to tour the island on our own. After we changed our plans and left the ship, the weather changed; the sun came out and shined so bright. We found a taxi and shared it with four other women who were a blast to be with. We laughed and talked the whole time. They shared our joy when we told them we were newlyweds.

We had a great time visiting the historic places and hearing about the government of the Bahamas. The driver took us to Atlantis, which is the grandest hotel and resort that I have ever seen. Large marble balls floating on water, light fixtures that are so ornate, moldings that appeared to be made of gold, and let's not forget, the casino. We stopped at the casino and dropped a few coins in the slot machines, trying to win that grand jackpot, but to no avail. We left a few dollars less than when we walked in, but who cares, we are on our honeymoon and having a great time. We played there for about an hour, went back to the taxi, and rode into the downtown district, which is not what I had envisioned. It was not as tropical and did not seem to live up to the picture of paradise that I had concocted in my head. Paula and I both had thought that when we arrived, there would be steel drum music playing, colorful birds everywhere, and everyone around singing and dancing. Well, it was not that way at all; maybe it was because of the weather or maybe that is not the way it is in real life, but nonetheless, we had a fabulous time. People on the island are quite different from people in the United States. We stopped in the world-famous straw market and walked what felt like hours, shopping for souvenirs to bring back and show our friends and family. I bought a large photo album, and Paula bought a smaller one; and when we compared information on what each had spent, I was the better shopper as we both had spent $20 for our albums. We shopped there for a while, went to eat, and then made our way back to the ship. This was such a great day even though we did not get to lie on the beach and soak up the sun.

The sun was going down, and we were about to set sail back for Florida, and as we watched Nassau fade in to the sunset, we went to our room and got ready for dinner. We had decided that Paula would wear her wedding dress and I would wear my tuxedo because we were going to have our picture taken later in the evening. Dinner was entertaining. Everyone was served, and when the meal was over, the waiters came around dancing and singing in a line while one man had a flaming dessert on his head.

After dinner, we went to the area of the ship that has a canvas painting of the grand staircase from the Titanic and had our photograph taken, Paula wearing her wedding dress and tiara on her head like a princess, holding my hand. I am so lucky to be married to such a beautiful woman. Later we went back to our stateroom, changed clothes, and then went up one floor to the casino on the ship. Paula played the slot machines; although winning small amounts, she would get so excited when the coins would fall into the metal tray and make the clinking sound. We played a short time, collected our winnings, and went to the top deck where we breathed in the fresh air and watched the moon glitter over the ocean. This is the most romantic thing I have ever experienced.

We sailed back to Florida and left the ship mostly sad because the fantasy was ending, and reality starting. We left Fort Lauderdale and headed northwest to Panama City, Florida. There we would stay a couple of days, relax, and grasp the idea that we are really married. Panama City was fun because I had never been there before and Paula had not been there for several years, so it was kind of new for both of us. After a couple of days, there we started the long drive back to Kentucky where we would go back to work and start living in the real world again.

We arrived at her house, got the luggage out of the car, went in, and went to bed. We were both worn out from the drive home. The next day, I had to go to my house that I lived in, get the rest of my clothes and some personal items, and move them in to Paula's house. We both had previously purchased houses not thinking of getting married as soon as we did. The house that I lived in is a little larger, but has a very small yard, which is not good for young children who need lots of room to run and play. We had discussed the idea to move into my house, but I explained that she had moved her boys around, and I thought that since they were established in this neighborhood with their friends, I would not want them to move, so we decided to live at her house. Brad, who was eleven years old; Logan, who was six years old; Paula; and I all got used to living with each other and our routine's fell into place pretty quick. Logan and I like to get up early, while she and Brad sleep late.

On the weekends that the boy's go to their dad's house, I let her sleep as late as she wants, so I watch television or meet a friend for breakfast.

We went back to work, shared our pictures and stories about our honeymoon with friends, and settled in to our new life together. It is different being in the same house with two young boys. It is an adjustment for all of us because each of us has different views on certain things. I get home most days before Paula, so I start dinner and start doing the daily chores that need to be done. She is very appreciative of this because her days can be long, and having to fix a meal for a family, start laundry, and general house cleaning can be hard; besides, my parents raised me to respect the fact that if a woman works outside the home, it is the husband's duty to help with household chores.

Holidays and Memories

Holidays are special for Paula, who is very sentimental about such things. She loves to decorate for all occasions, putting out various items for each holiday to bring cheer to the house. We got through Halloween, Thanksgiving, and now comes Christmas.

One morning, the first week of December 2007, as she was getting ready for work, she called me into the bathroom to show me a bruise on her left breast. I asked her how it happened, and she explained that she did not know. I thought one of our pets had possibly jumped on her while she was sitting, causing it to bruise. We decided to keep a close watch on it to see if it went away, but approximately two weeks went by and the bruise was getting larger, and she was beginning to feel some pain. December 26, 2007, she contacted the doctor to get an appointment because she hated to disturb him during the holiday. By now, her breast was starting to enlarge; it felt warm to the touch and was bruised beyond compare to any bruise I had ever seen. We went for an office visit. At this time, he diagnosed her with an infection and put her on antibiotics, which seemed to help at first; but then a few days later, the symptom regained strength, and by now the pain was unbearable for her. He also prescribed pain medication for her, which did not help much. Two weeks later, he performed an ultrasound of her breast, which showed no abnormality. He then started another round of antibiotics. Later she was referred to a diagnostic facility to have a more detailed ultrasound, which also did not show any abnormality.

Now the skin had started to look worse, more heat, pain, and now texturing of the skin to resemble the appearance of an orange peel and severe bruising. How she was tolerating the pain, only she and God knows. After nothing being resolved, she was referred to an infectious disease specialist with whom we met. She was examined by the doctor who then stated that it could be one of several types of infection or IBC. When I asked what IBC is, she said, "That is inflammatory breast carcinoma." I remarked, "Cancer?" And she said, "Yes, but it is the lowest on the list." I don't think that is what this is.

By now, I am wondering why not treat for the worst, and then if that is not the problem, treat for infection. This doctor starts her on more antibiotics, and we leave going home so Paula can lie down and rest later on. Her sister and I had been looking on the internet about this IBC and were comparing notes without Paula's knowledge, and she seemed to present all but one of the symptoms.

After that course of antibiotics, nothing is working. In the meantime, I had been out of town for a few days, during which time I contacted a friend of mine who is a radiologist and explained the situation to him. He told me to bring her to his office on Monday and let him get her an appointment with a doctor who would do a biopsy. When I returned on Friday to meet Paula for lunch, she was in so much pain.

She called the surgeon to see if he would call the hospital for her to get a shot to help ease the pain. When we arrived at his office to get the prescription to take to the hospital for the shot, he wanted to see her to which I explained she was in too much pain to get out and come into his office. He walked with me to the car where she waited and coaxed her to come in and let him look at her breast, which she did. He stated that he would set up for a biopsy, and I told him that she had an appointment on Monday, and he wanted to know with whom, so I told him. He asked his secretary to get the other doctor on the phone, and they spoke about this at length, to which he told me that the other doctor wanted to talk with me. My friend told me to go ahead and let him do the biopsy.

Heartbreak

Monday, February 18, 2008, came, and we went to the hospital for the procedure, knowing all the while in the back of my mind my new bride has cancer. Her sister Cathy, Aunt Jonell, and Uncle Dwayne were with us for support. After a while, the doctor came out, took us into a small room, and notified us he was sure it was cancer but had sent a sample to pathology for verification. He wanted to see us in his office on Tuesday.

Tuesday morning, February 19, we met in his office to hear the heartbreaking news: "Yes, it is Cancer". Inflammatory breast carcinoma is rare and very aggressive. It starts as a small bruise, begins to worsen with heat, tenderness, and a lot of pain. The skin will begin to have the appearance of an orange peel. I felt as if someone had placed a million pounds on my shoulders and pulled all of the oxygen from my lungs. We cried together, and he stated that he wanted her to see an oncologist and made an appointment for that afternoon. Before we left his office, he asked if he could pray with us. When we met with the oncologist in Bowling Green, I did not feel comfortable with her, as she had treated my mother who had died some years before due to throat cancer. Paula's sister Cathy said that we had to contact MD Anderson Cancer Center in Houston, Texas, because they are the best in cancer treatment in the nation. We will do what it takes to get her better because she has already promised me fifty years of marriage. The short trip back home was quiet because at this point, no one knows what to say. After all of the years I have spent working on the road, coming to Bowling Green, and finding the love of my life, my soul mate, I stood a good chance to loose her to this dreadful disease. When we got home, her sister Cathy came by, and we immediately got on line to MD Anderson Cancer Center. I completed a self-referral form and contacted the physician who had preformed the biopsy to see if he would call and refer her as well. The next day, we were contacted by someone at MDACC. We answered a few questions and were told that we would be contacted by someone else within twenty-four hours.

February 22, we received a call and answered more questions, and the party on the end of the line asked, "When can you be here?" To which we replied, "Whenever we need to." Paula's brother-in-law Donnie met with me at the travel agency to make reservations for the flight and hotel because I had never done this before. Paula's sisters, Cathy and Edwina, and niece Natasha went to Belmont Baptist Church in Morgantown, Kentucky, on Sunday morning to worship with us. Paula was anointed by Brother Embry and the deacons of the church. I had a feeling that God would make everything right, and this would be a quick treatment and our new life together would begin as planned.

The flight was going to be a nerve-racking experience for me as I have never been on an airplane before and was not sure about it. Even though Paula had never flown before either, she asked me before we were married of what I would do if she would not marry me if I would not fly to our honeymoon destination; just to get my reaction. My reply was, "It has been nice knowing you, I will not fly." But when she was diagnosed with cancer, my remark was, "I will be the first one on the plane." It is because it is a fifteen-hour drive to Houston from Bowling Green. I knew in my heart she could not stand the pain of jarring around in a car for that long, no matter how many stops we made.

February 27, we left for the airport in Nashville, Tennessee, to embark on a new but not so exciting journey as we had done in the past. We woke this morning to snow on the ground. This journey would determine how much time I would have to spend with my love and best friend. Donnie and Cathy drove us with Bradley and Logan to the airport to say our goodbyes. We would be gone approximately ten days, which about broke her heart as she had not spent that much time away from Bradley and Logan except when we went on our honeymoon. I was standing at the windows watching workers spray de-icing solution on a plane when this man walked up and started a conversation with me by asking how I was doing. I explained to him that I was nervous about flying, and he eased my mind somewhat. You see, he was a pilot who had flown to Nashville from Houston the previous day and was helpful with information about the pilot who would be flying us to Houston. As it turned out, he would be the pilot flying the plane. It is my belief that God had sent this man to comfort me and help me with my fear of flying. We boarded the plane, me in front, as I had promised to be the first to get on. We walked to the rear of the plane and took our seats, and as time drew closer to departing, I was getting more nervous, so I took something to calm my nerves, which did not take effect until we were airborne. We landed in Houston, and when I started off of the plane, the pilot was waiting to greet me to see how I had tolerated the flight. He also introduced us to the other pilot whose father was a doctor at MDACC. We picked up our rental car, drove to the hotel, and settled in for the evening. All of this was so new to both of us; I felt a little awkward not knowing where to go and what to do when I got there.

Day's at the Clinic

February 28, we boarded a shuttle van to the Mays Clinic where we were given a schedule of her appointments to which there were many. It was one appointment after another with a short time in between to get from one place to the next. There was no time to eat or even get a snack. The first day is always busy for any patient who is diagnosed with an illness such as cancer. It can drain all of your energy, not only the patient, but also any person that is accompanying the patient. That afternoon, we were waiting in an exam room when Dr. Massimo Cristofinilli came in and spoke with us. He looked at Paula's breast without touching her. He showed the most respect and concern for Paula, patted her on the leg, and said, "We're going to take care of you." To hear that lifted so much from me as I knew in my heart that he was telling the truth. They would take care of her. Dr. Cristofinilli is the head of the breast center and treated a young woman with IBC. She lost her battle with cancer, and he carries her wedding picture in his lab coat pocket every day as a reminder of this terrible cancer.

Then we met Dr. Eleni Andreopoulou, the lady doctor who would be treating Paula. She told us of the chemotherapy treatments and how it would affect her. It would turn out to be twenty-four weeks, twelve weeks of one chemo drug Taxol, then followed up by twelve weeks of the real bad chemo known as FEC. Some people have told us that is called "The Red Devil" because of its color and the side effects it brings. She is also receiving Herceptin, a special drug that works to fill holes in the cell structure as I understand it. This will continue for one year.

Friday, February 29, 8:00 a.m., we are met by a lady who works in clinical trials and asked if Paula would participate in a study for this type of breast cancer. The lady of whom I do not know her name explained that not many patients participate in this study for one reason or another. I suppose it is the pain or the lack of information that is available to the patient. After all this is a study that will be ongoing for months, possibly years. Paula agreed to have a punch biopsy and would have to be back in the clinic on Monday. She had more tests and blood draws. I felt so sorry for her having to endure all of the needles, mammograms, PET scans, CAT scans, and ultrasounds. But tomorrow would be better. It is Saturday, and we have plans to go to Galveston. Another new adventure and another memory. Paula is all about memories. Sometimes, she will say, "You know what we're doing? We're making a memory." Now I understand why because we don't know how much time we have to spend with loved ones.

Saturday, March 1, we drive to Galveston, Texas. It is about fifty miles south of Houston. Going down Highway 59 South, we started seeing oil refineries and were in awe of all of the storage tanks. Being from a small town in Kentucky, we don't get the opportunity to see a lot of things like this. We arrived not knowing where we were going or what there was to do. So we started down Seawall Boulevard, looking at the ocean, souvenir shops, various restaurants, and hotels. We drove up and down the boulevard, stopping at different shops for Paula to go into and find treasures to bring back home. We must have stopped at every souvenir shop on the strip. All I was interested in was collecting sand and some shells from the beach. The three times I have been to the ocean now, I have collected sand and shells. It's a cheap hobby, not to mention, my concept of a memory. We decided that this would be the perfect place to be spontaneous and check into a hotel for the night, which was just what we did. No change of clothes, no makeup for her, and no toothbrushes. That is what I like to do, to be spontaneous. We checked in and went back out for some more sightseeing, ate, walked on the beach (which is not real pretty); but being with my wife, I never really noticed until Sunday morning when I walked across the street to the oceanfront. I met several nice people with whom I talked and explained why we were there. Most of them said they would pray for her and keep us in their thoughts.

Sunday morning, Paula woke up, and we had breakfast at a pancake house, shopped a little more, and headed back to Houston. One more memory. We had to rest after we got back to the hotel we were staying at because tomorrow is more tests and meeting with a breast surgeon. Monday morning, March 3, after the round of tests, we had time to grab a quick bite, then on to meet with Dr. Anthony Lucci. He spoke with us about how he would perform the surgery and what the results would be, as well as any complications. About six months after she has completed all of the chemotherapy treatments is when he will schedule the bilateral mastectomy. I am feeling confident with all of the doctors and health care professionals who are taking care of her, but I still know that God is in control and there is no way he will let anything happen to her.

Tuesday, March 4, Paula has no tests today and no meetings with doctors, so it is a free day. We drove north of Houston to a town called Old Spring. It is an old town where the houses on the main street have been turned into novelty shops. Colorful buildings and warm weather can be such good therapy for the soul and help to forget your problems for a little while. There was even a shop that specializes in items for pets. We spent a lot of time in this shop looking around. I have a dog, Maggie, a Jack Russell beagle mix and Paula has Riley, a cockapoo. Her dog looks after Maggie since he is only three years and Maggie is about fifteen years old. When we go to Texas, we leave them with Joelyn, a lady that sits with pets, so we know they are well taken care of and that is one less worry.

Wednesday, March 5, starts at 6:30 a.m. with more tests, scans of her brain and ovaries, ultrasound, and MRI. She is a little nervous about going into the MRI machine as she gets claustrophobic when she is in tight spots. We are in the Mays Clinic until 9:00 p.m. The ultrasound showed some type of tumors in the right breast, lymph nodes, and duodenum.

Thursday, March 6, Dr. Andreopoulou's physician assistant Pam Vranas came in to discuss the results of the tests. The bone scan showed some abnormality in the left leg, but she said not to worry. She also informed us that they were waiting on the results from other tests to come back. She tried to get an upper GI scheduled but with no luck. We went back to the waiting room for them to call her in for the punch biopsy. When they called her back, I moved to another chair and overheard a couple talking to the same clinical trial lady that we had talked to about having the same procedure done. Her husband was not happy about her going through this without having access to the results (which there are no results) as it is an ongoing study and how it would not benefit her. She refused to participate, so I walked around and explained that my wife was here with a rare breast cancer and was in a lot of pain and was proceeding with this procedure so that maybe it would help someone else in the future. She asked the receptionist to call the trial nurse and did choose to participate.

After having four holes the size of small pencils punched in her bruised and very tender breast, it was time to start upstairs for Paula's first chemotherapy treatment. Paula and I had asked Dr. Eleni if it would be possible to get some of her treatments at home because getting chemo as often as she was going to have to, there would be no way we could make a weekly trip to Houston. She explained that she would contact the doctor in Bowling Green to see if she would be willing to give the same course of medicine that they would use in Texas. It was approximately 6:30 p.m. when we arrived, and they got started soon after. The room we were in was nice, with a television. The first drug, Herceptin, went very well; but when the nurse started the Taxol, we had been told of side effects to watch for, and Paula started getting a backache. I immediately called for the nurse, and she came in with a tray of medicines and informed us that she was having an allergic reaction to it. She started pushing Benadryl in the IV and Paula got very sleepy, but her back quit hurting. We were there until 9:10 p.m. that evening, then had to drive back to the hotel.

Friday, March 7, is the first time we got to visit with the pain management doctors. They were very nice and understanding to her pain level. These doctors came in and evaluated the pain Paula was having and started her on Lyrica and other medications for the pain, which was caused by the nerve endings. We are supposed to fly back to Nashville tomorrow, but there is heavy snow, so we delayed the flight until Sunday.

FRIENDS AND FAMILY HELP

Going back and forth to Houston can be very expensive. We have struggled with finances since this all began, but thanks to the utility company where Paula works, several employees where I work, and her family holding benefits, raffles, bake sales, and different fund-raisers, we have been blessed with enough money to make several trips.

Had it not been for the generosity of these and others, of which there to many to mention, this would not have been possible. There were also people who donated money for Paula at a family-oriented music club in Morgantown, Kentucky, where Paula's Sister Cathy plays on Friday nights. People go to hear the down-home country sounds and some travel from as far as Tennessee. The Rose family who owns this club held a benefit, and people crowded into the building to listen to music, play games, and bid on various items that had been donated. There were cakes that were auctioned for as much as $200. One man drove from Glasgow, Kentucky, which is quite far from Morgantown and offered his services to be the auctioneer. This benefit was a great success especially after we found out that an insurance company offered to match the amount of money raised. We are going to be home for a couple of weeks, trying to get back to normal routine. Paula still has some pain but not as bad as it was because of the pain medication. Now she is taking OxyContin, and Oxycodone. I am afraid that if she takes too much, she might get addicted to this, but I guess the doctors know what they are doing. At night when we sit down to eat, Logan will give the blessing and always thanks God for healing his mother. It is so sweet that a six-year-old child can believe that strongly in the powers of God.

March 25, we are back at Mays Clinic to meet with Dr. Peter Pisters, a surgical oncologist. He is going to schedule a procedure to see what the tumor is that is in her duodenum. He said that he thinks that it is a GIST (gastrointestinal stromal tumor). He is going to contact her oncologist to advise her of when procedure will be performed to see exactly what it is and send a piece of it for a biopsy. They are more intent with the breast cancer right now than they are with this tumor, although the tumor is somewhat of a priority. Thursday, March 27, Paula went into surgery to have a portacath implanted in her upper chest in front of her right shoulder. The portacath will give the nurses access to her veins without having to have an IV placed in her arm each time chemo is administered. Dr. Irvin Brown did this surgery, and everything went very well. We went back to the hotel, and Paula slept well tonight. Paula had to be at the hospital on Friday, March 28, to have the scope inserted in her throat to check the tumor in her duodenum. The procedure started on time and was over in about fifteen minutes. The doctor came out and informed me that there was some leftover food in her stomach so the anesthesiologist stopped the procedure. We would have to come back on Monday to try again.

Monday, March 28, we are back for a second try at the procedure. This time he was able to remove a piece of it and sent it to the pathologist to determine what it is. After resting for a while, we leave for home at 8:45 p.m.

April has been a calm month, no trips to Texas, just time to adjust to being home and becoming a closer family. We still have difficulty sometimes, but no family is without problems. Ours is mainly the discipline of school homework with Bradley. He is so intelligent, but he has trouble in some of his classes. He is very artistic and creates outstanding stories of fantasy. If his energy went to homework like it does his drawings and writing, he would have no problems at all. Logan is in the second grade. On most days, he does his homework. He too is very intelligent and loves video games. He is a good boy who tries very hard to please everyone.

Once again, we return to Texas for some more tests and another series of chemo treatments. While we are in Bowling Green, Paula receives treatments from the oncologist that we visited when we found out that she had cancer. The only reason Paula sees her is that she follows the exact orders as prescribed by Dr. Eleni. Pam, Dr. Eleni's PA came into the room and told us that everything is going well. After Pam left, we smiled at one another, so glad to hear the news that everything is going well means so much. Dr. Eleni came in and gave us the news that the cancer is 50 percent gone. I felt as if this large weight had been lifted off of my shoulders. There are five stages of cancer, and when Paula first got there, she was at stage 4. I got the feeling that the doctor did not expect this kind of result.

A New Friend

Tonight we are in the hotel room, and Paula got a call from Cathy. She told Paula that her housekeeper, Zeljka (pronounced "Zeeka"), had been told by her doctor that she too had breast cancer. Zeljka had lost her husband a few years earlier to cancer, and she was very scared. She has two children (both boy's) like Paula. Cathy told her she needed to contact MD Anderson to see about getting treatment. After I got her the information to do a self-referral, she was accepted as a patient and had to figure out how she was going to get the money to get there. Fortunately, another lady she works for helped with the finances and travel plans. When she arrived at MD Anderson Cancer Center, she came to have the same physician that Paula has. One day, Zeljka is with the doctor and has Paula's name on a piece of paper, which Dr. Eleni noticed, and asked her, "How do you know this woman?" Zeljka told her of being from Bowling Green and being Paula's sister housekeeper. Dr. Andreopoulou thought it was odd that she would be treating two women from the same town who knew one another. Paula nor myself had ever met Zeljka, but we both felt a kinship with her. It turned out that she was staying at the same hotel as we were, but the next day would be the strangest of all.

I had driven Paula to the clinic, gone back to the hotel to park the car, and walked back to the clinic. I stepped into the elevator and pushed the button to the fifth floor when the eighth-floor light came on. There were several people on the elevator, so I made a comment about both lights coming on. This dark-haired lady told me that she had pushed the eighth-floor button.

When I looked at her, I could see the bandage where she recently had a portable catheter put in her chest for chemotherapy treatments and heard her voice. I asked her, "Are you from Bowling Green?" She looked at me like I was stalking her, then acknowledged that she was. At that time, I told her who I was.

We got off of the elevator on the fifth floor, hugged, and talked for a moment. Paula and I thought she had gone home that morning because she stays only the time needed for appointments then goes home. At this time, Paula had not met Zeljka as she had been called in for her appointment. It must be real terrifying for her being in a strange city alone and not having anything to occupy your spare time away from the clinic.

Now we are into June of 2008, and we are headed back to Houston. This time, Brad and Logan went with us. I thought Logan would be scared on the plane, but it was Brad that got really nervous when the plane started down the runway. The plane was so crowded that none of us could sit together, which upset Paula. She wanted to sit with them so that they would not be scared. Logan loved it. The next day, we went to the clinic for an appointment with the oncologist. When Dr. Eleni came into the room, she was so glad to see that we had brought them. She kissed Logan on the cheek, smiled the whole time, and made sure that they knew how important it was that their mother is going to be fine.

The time we spent in Texas was good for them, so now they know what the clinic and hospital looks like. Brad thought it would be old and dismal, but now he sees that it is modern and clean.

July 16 is here, and we are back. Today, Paula is scheduled for more tests. Today is the longest that we have ever had to wait, five hours to see Dr. Lucci. Paula can get a scheduled date for the mastectomy. We have to wait until September. She just wants to get it over with. While we were waiting, I told Paula that the first trip was the most lonesome that I had ever been. Not being away from home, but going to a cancer hospital and going into the unknown as I had no idea how long I would have her in my life. We had dinner and drove to Kemah, Texas, an amusement area south of Houston. At this point in time, I feel as though Paula needs all of the time she can get to have as much fun as she can because of the effects from the treatments. We walked on the boardwalk and had fun for a while. Paula is so tired as the chemo treatments are starting to wear her down. She doesn't sleep well at night, but then neither do I. By now her hair is starting to come out. She wakes up, and there are large amounts of hair on her pillow. She is starting to get depressed about this a little, but it is to be expected. She actually let Logan help her cut her long strings of hair, so that he would not feel so bad about her having really short hair or none at all.

THE NEWS

July 17 is the day that we have been waiting for. We met with Dr. Eleni, and Paula has brought her a sundress from Bowling Green. When the physician assistant came in, she asked if we wanted good news or GOOD NEWS. The PET scan shows no cancer at all; IT IS GONE!!! I have had this load lifted from me, and I know Paula feels the same. When we leave the clinic, we will celebrate. We went to a hamburger restaurant. When someone has cancer, sometimes a small thing is a large accomplishment. What a celebration. I believe it was the best hamburger I have ever eaten. But it doesn't matter. My wife is with me. The other good news is that we don't have to come back for a while.

Back home, we try to go through our daily routine: get the boys off to school, go to work, and come home. I try to do as much as I can to help, but Paula is headstrong that she is not going to let chemo get her completely down, but she gets so tired. I love her so much that I want her to rest and save her strength so she can tolerate treatments better. She is such a fighter.

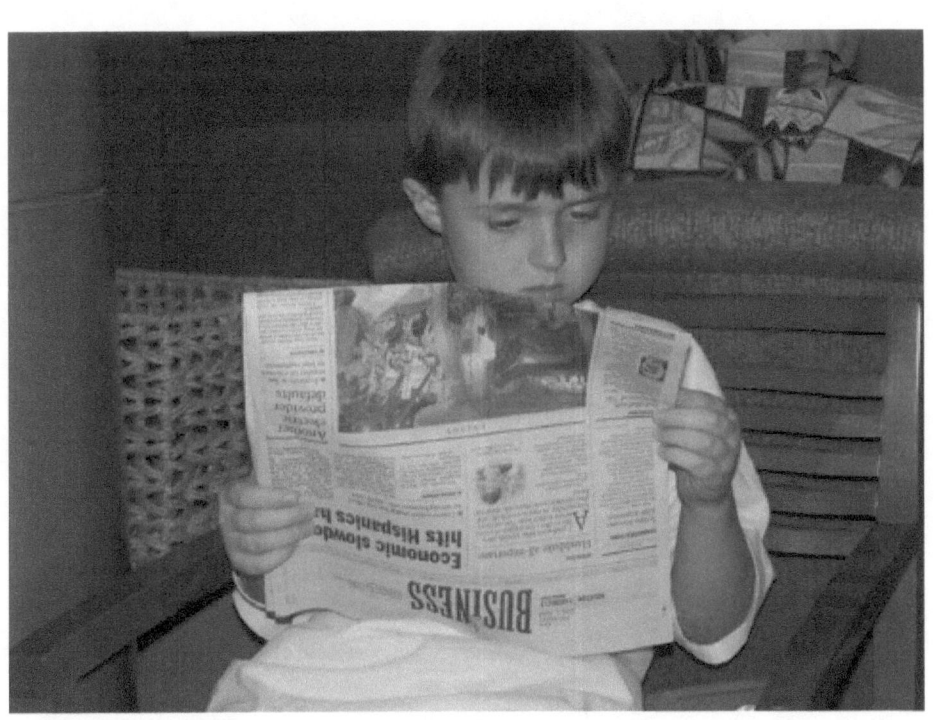

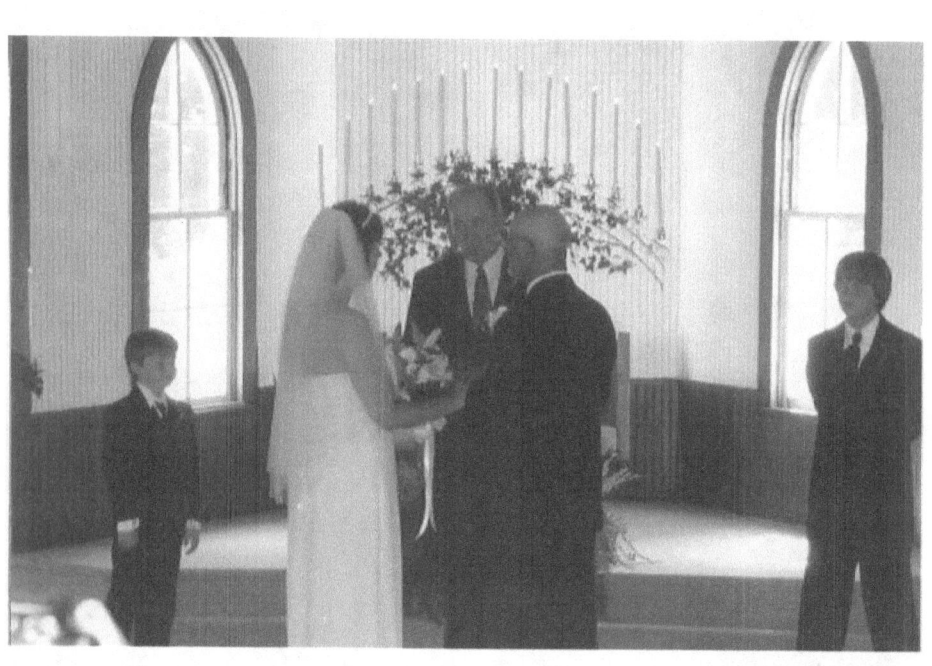

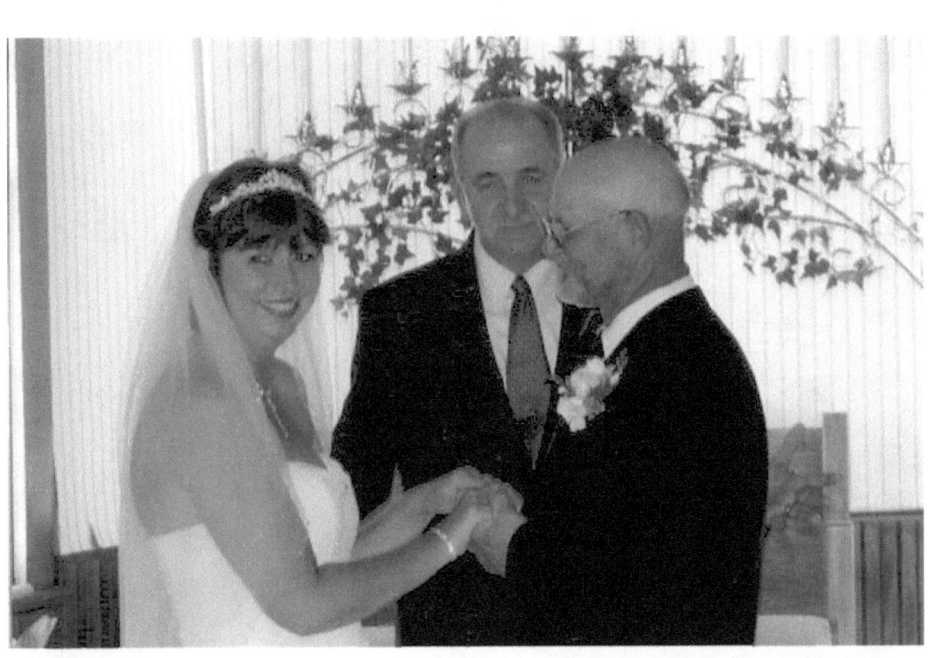

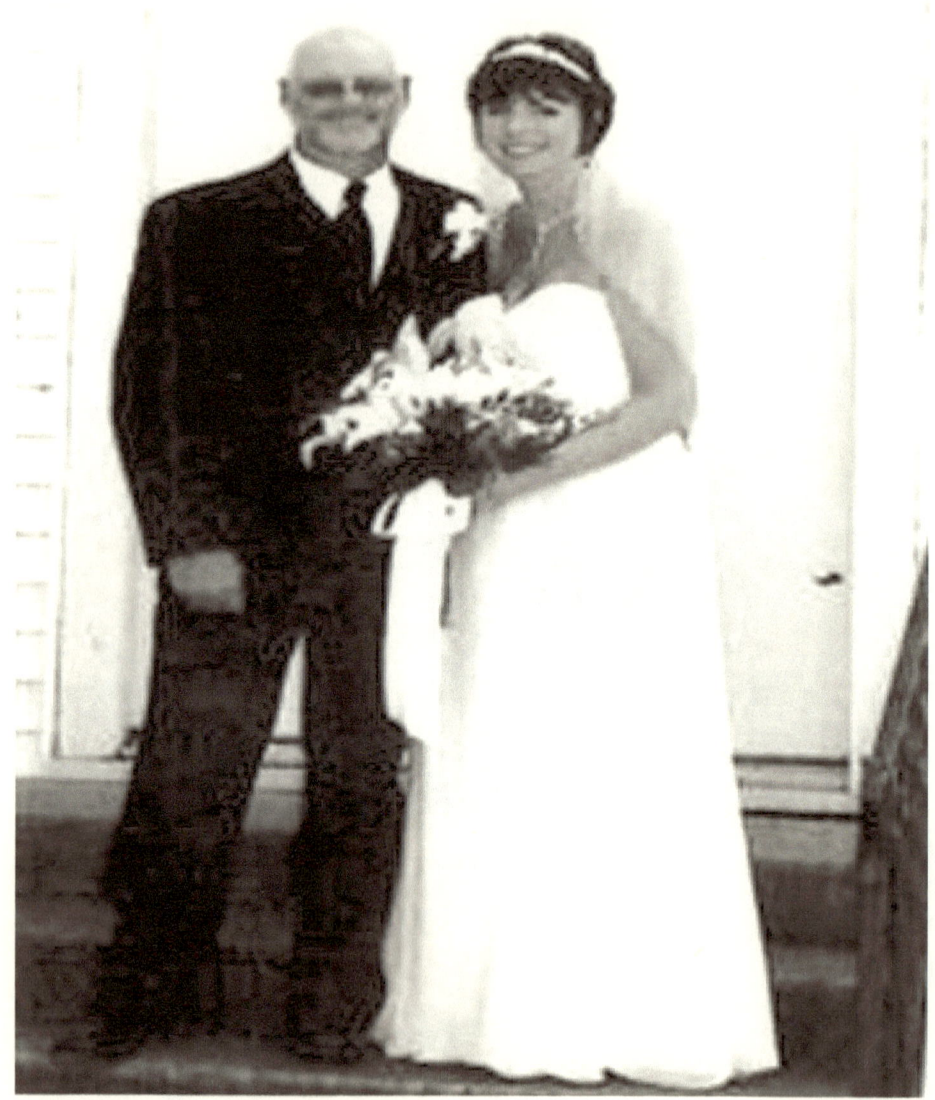

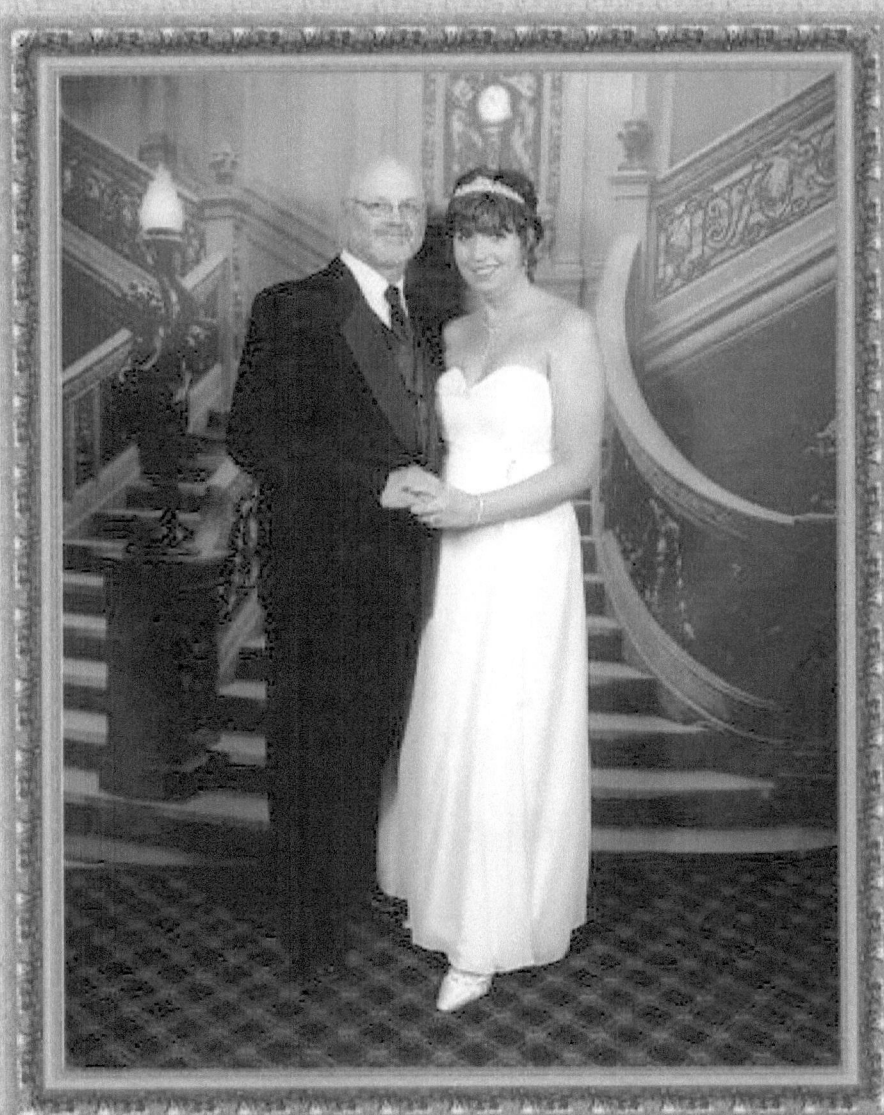

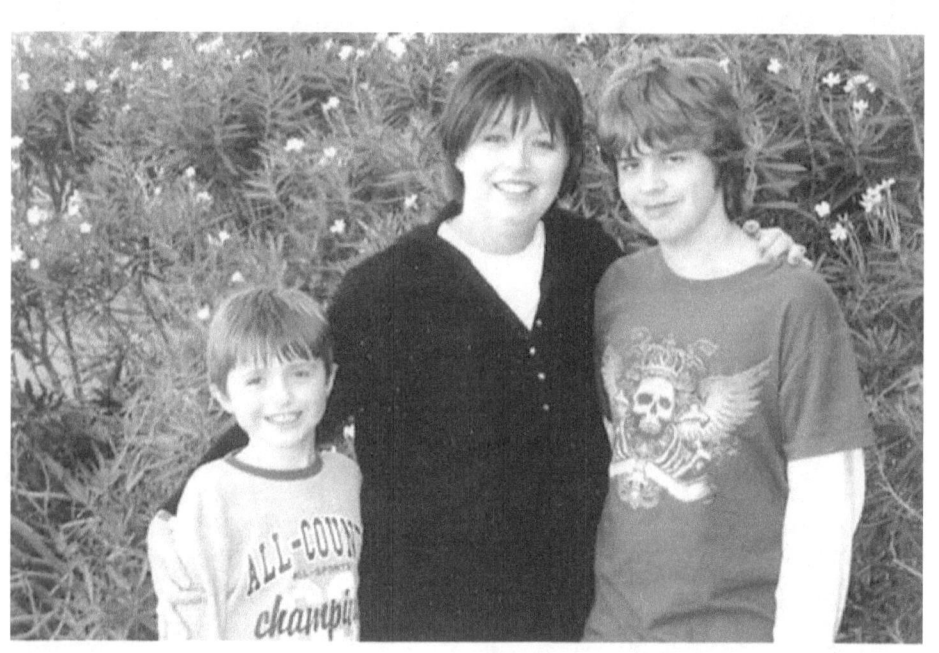

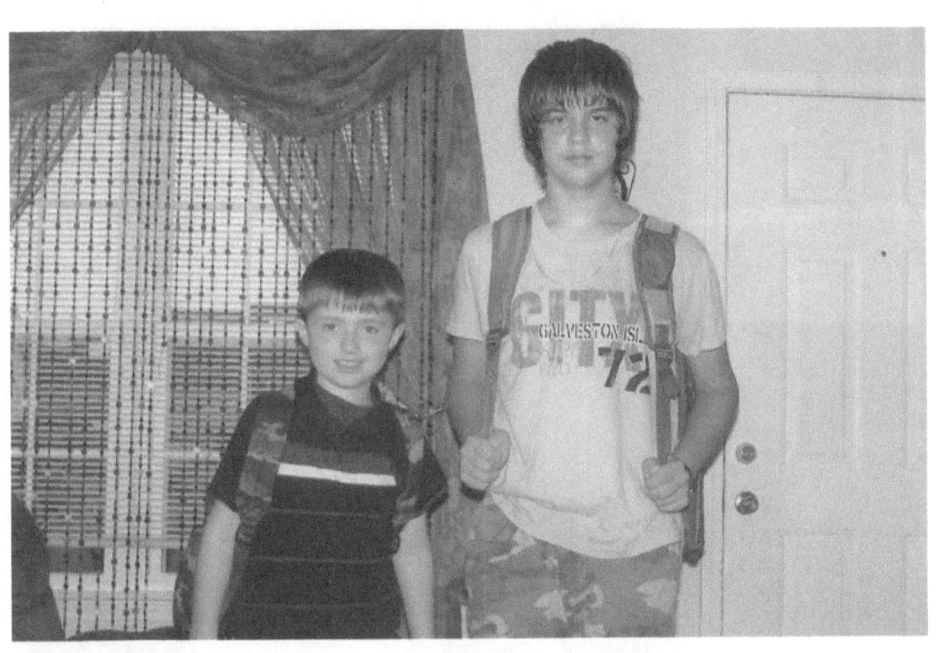

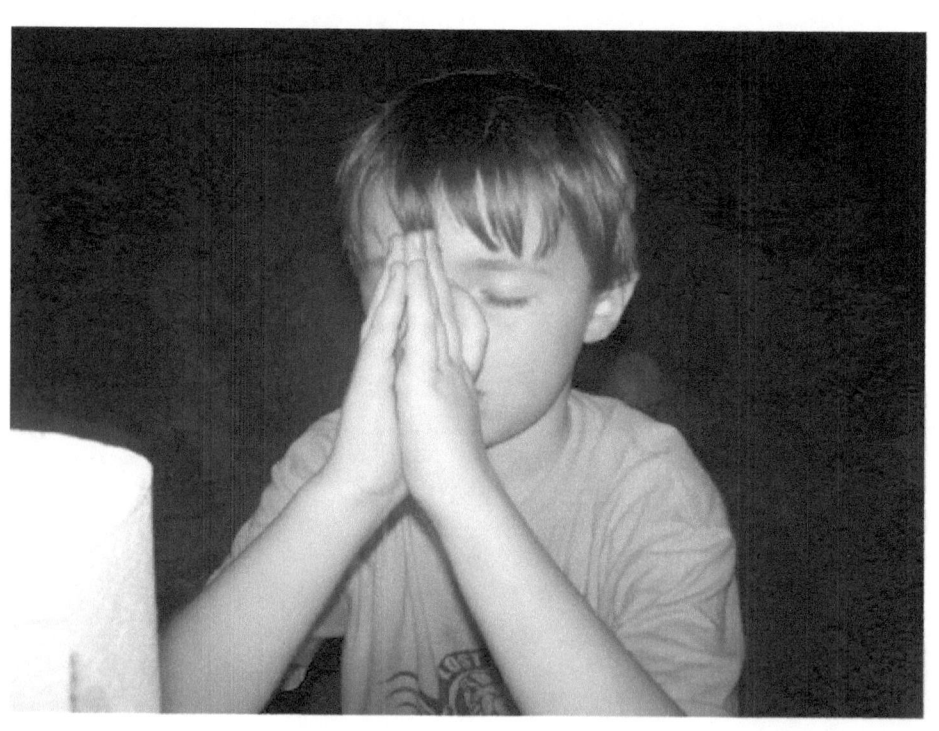

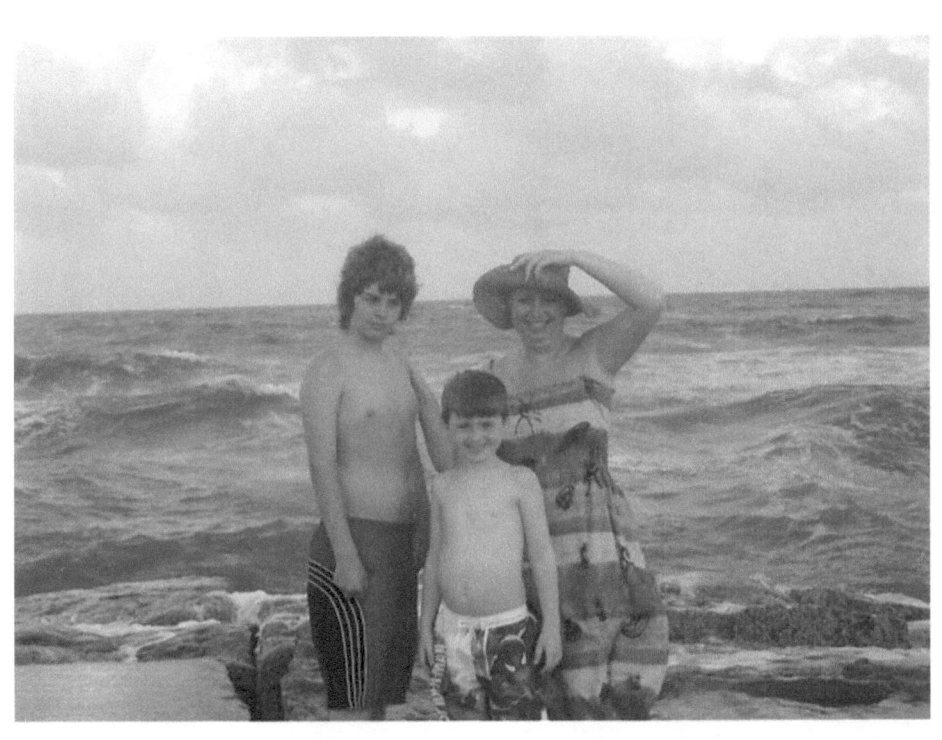

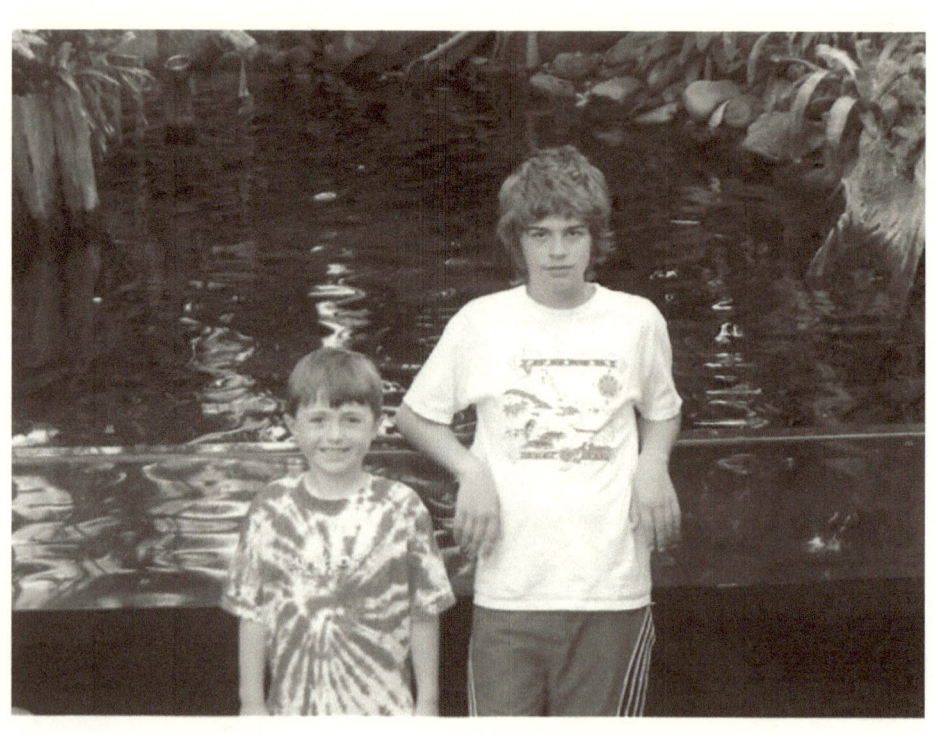

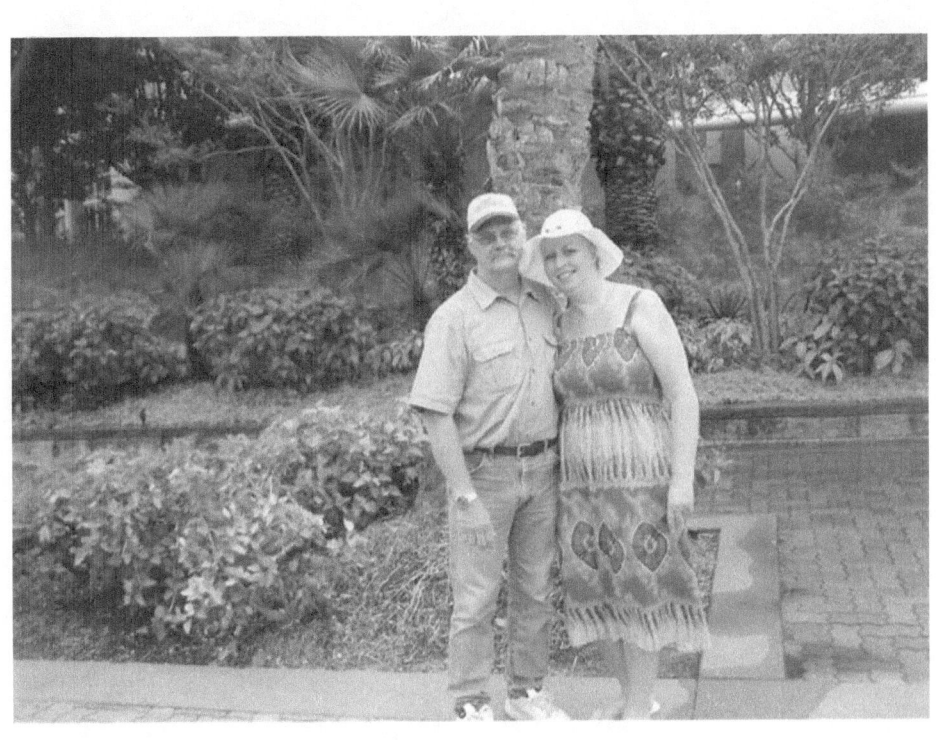

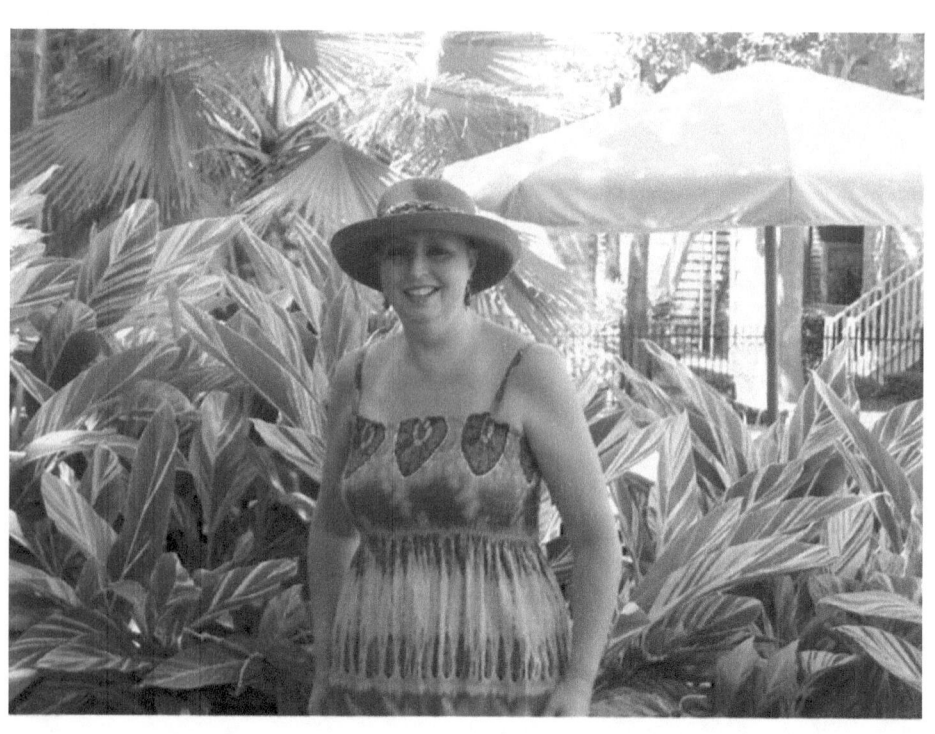

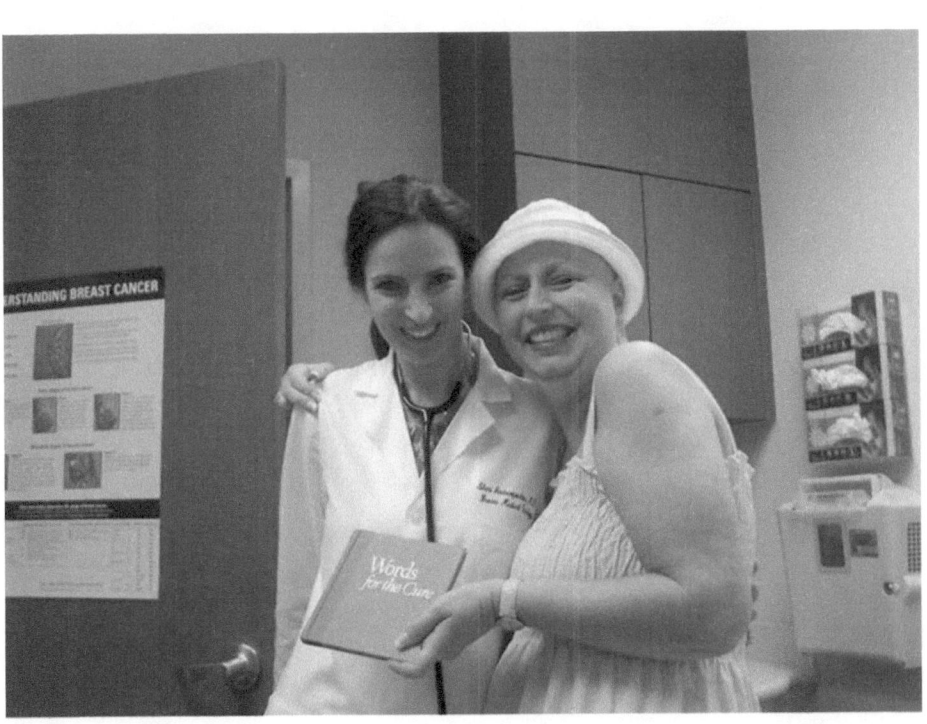

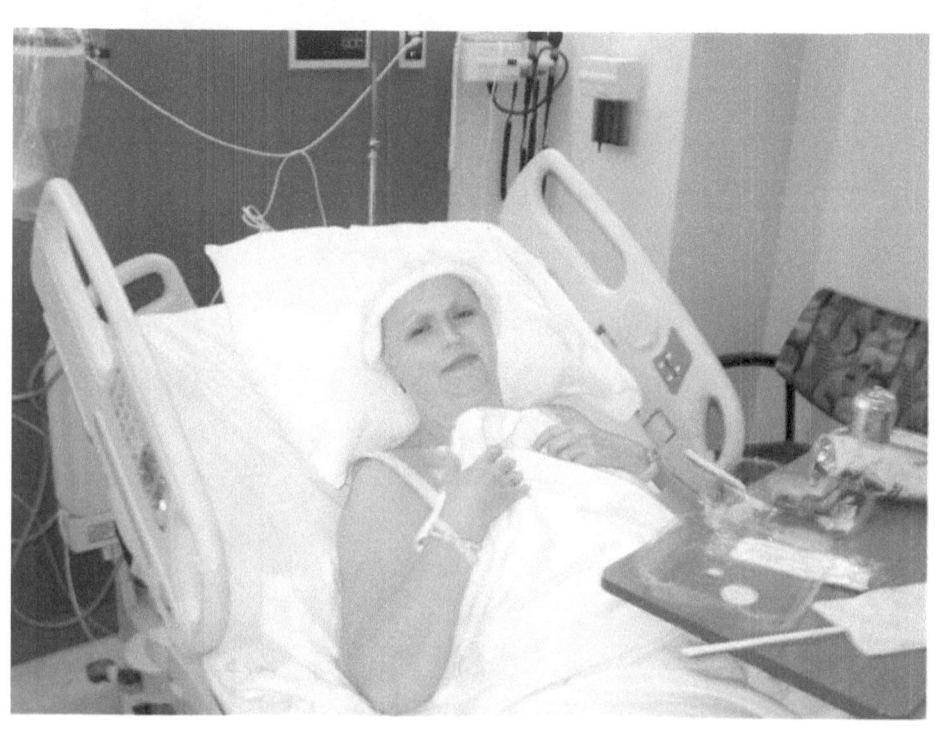

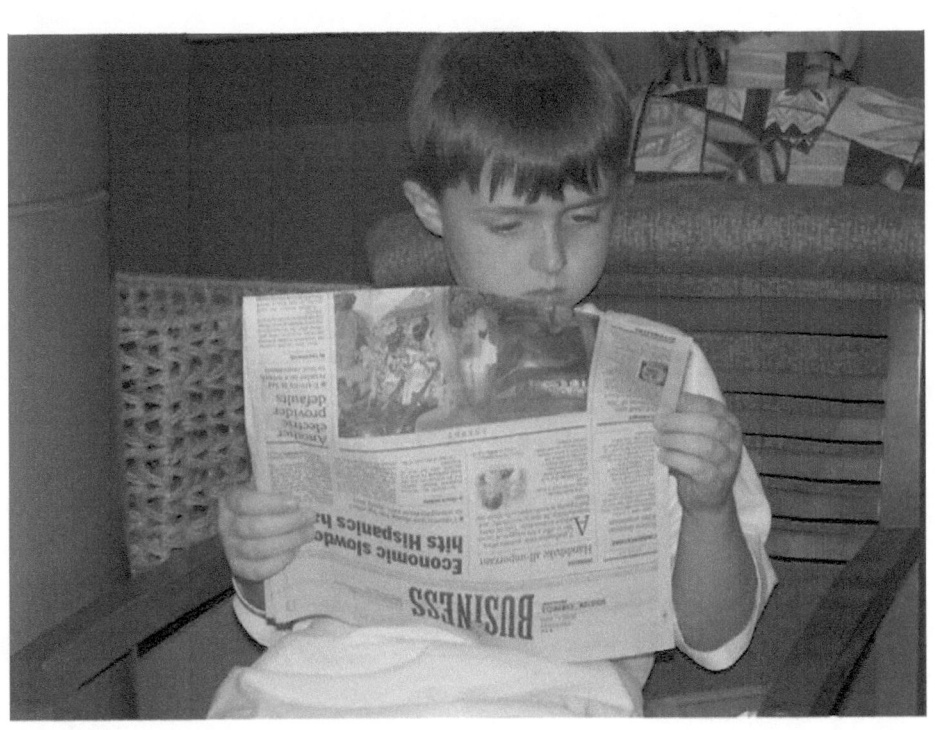

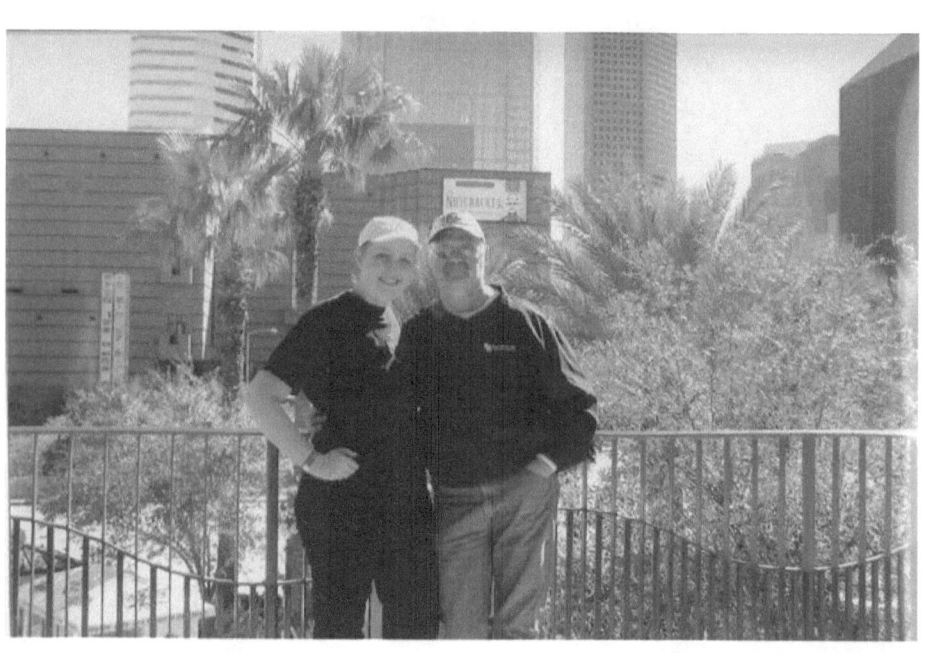

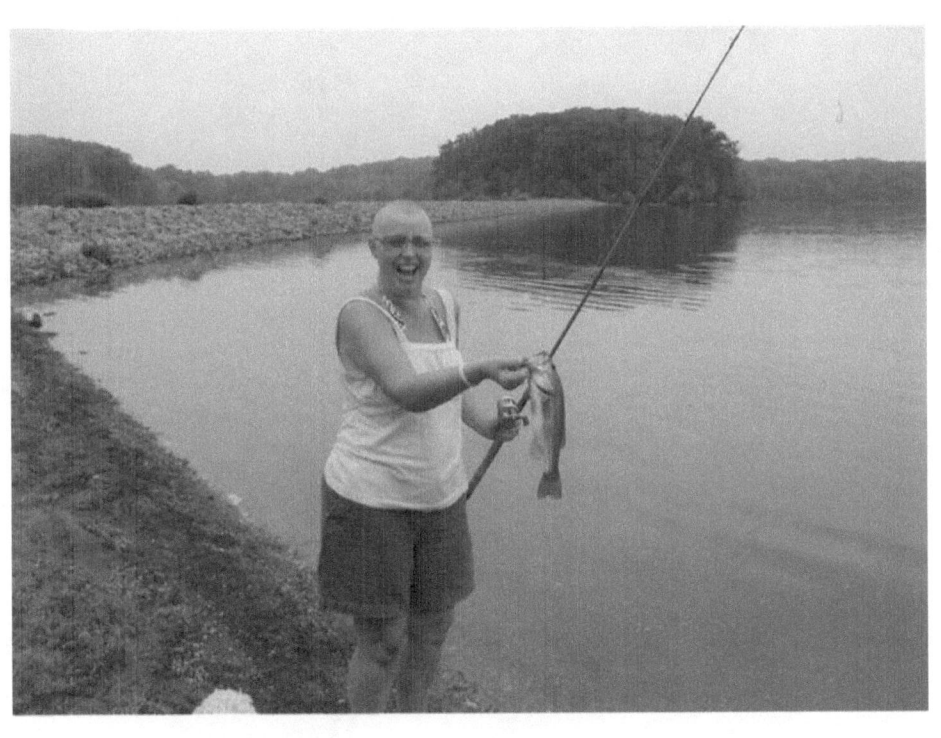

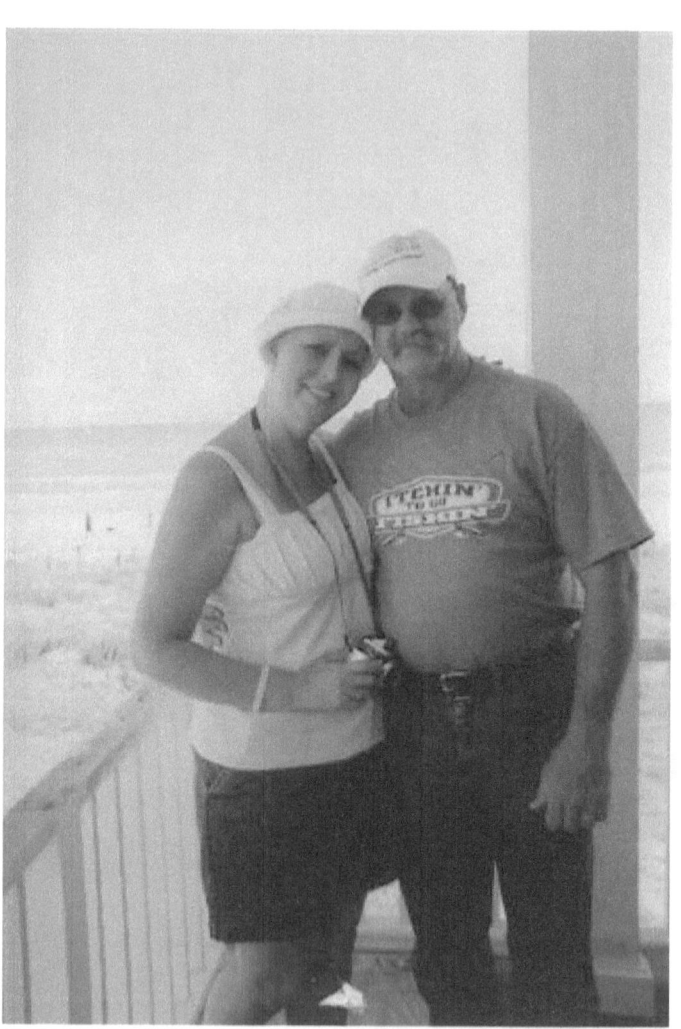

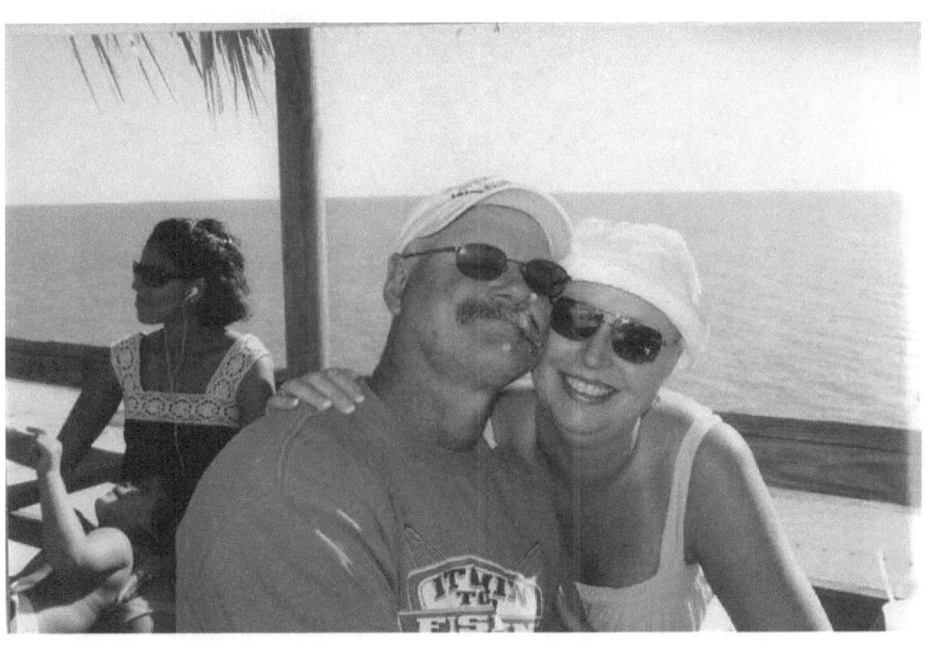

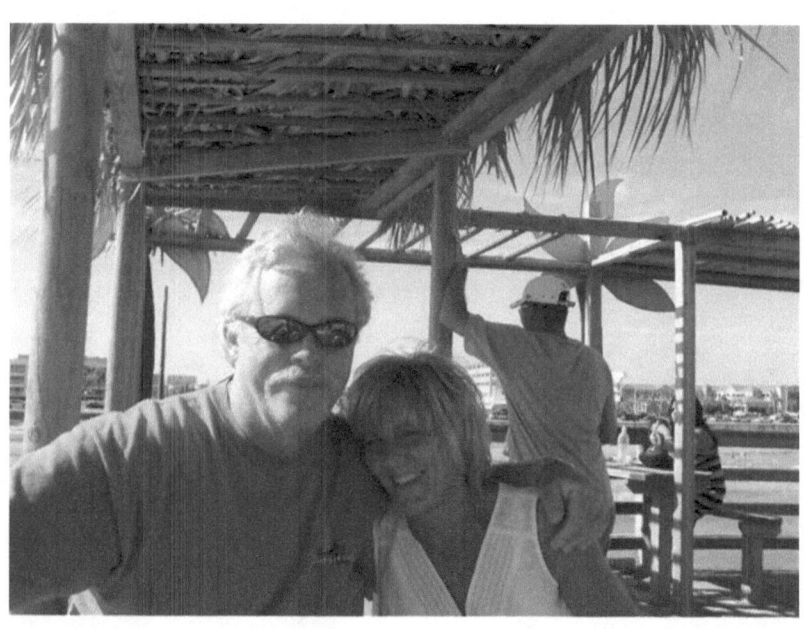

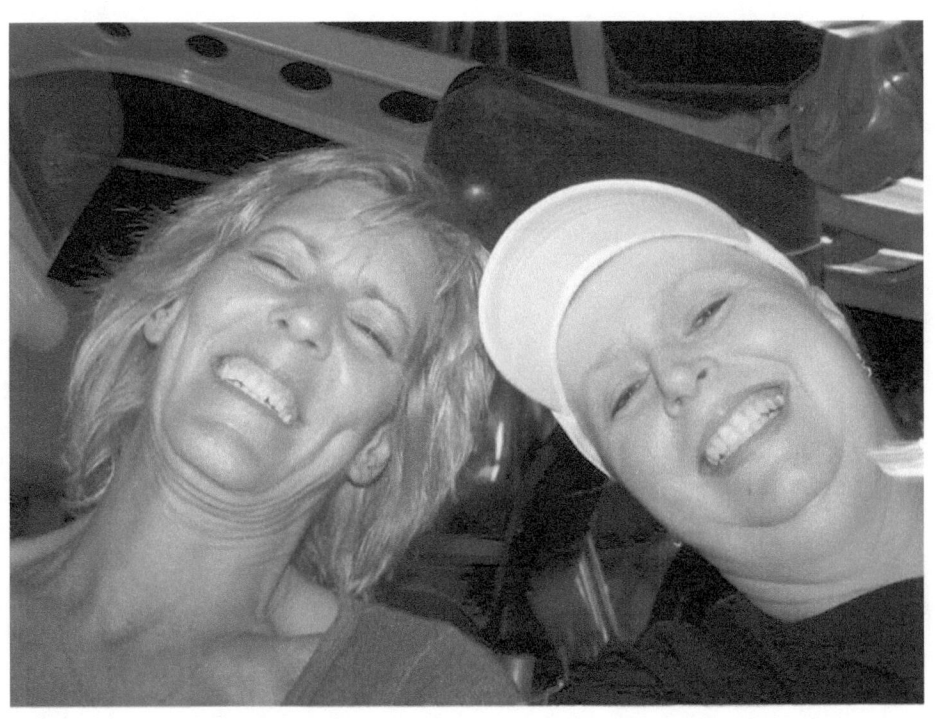

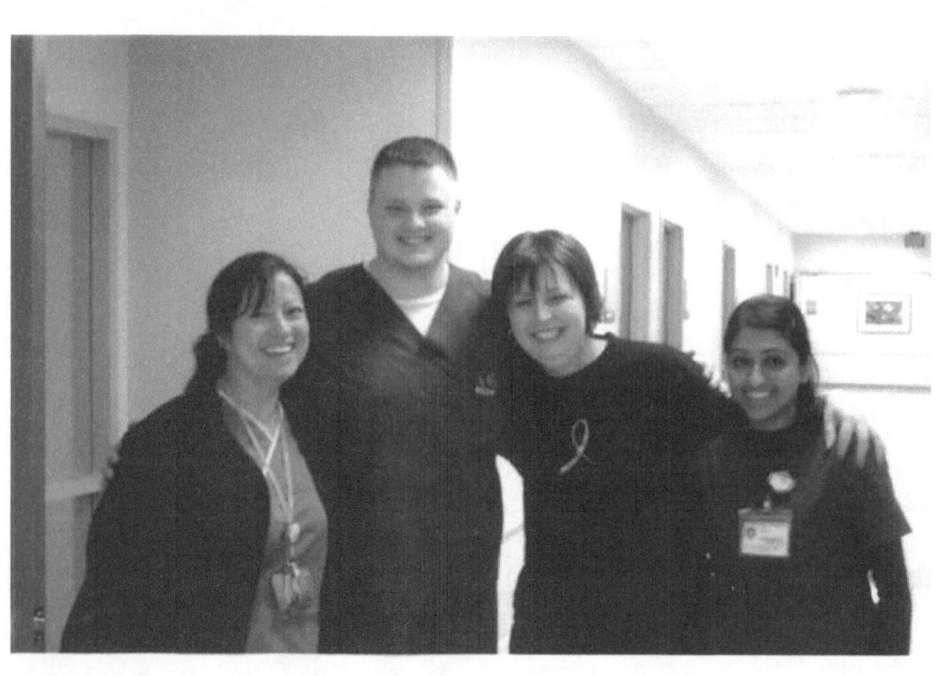

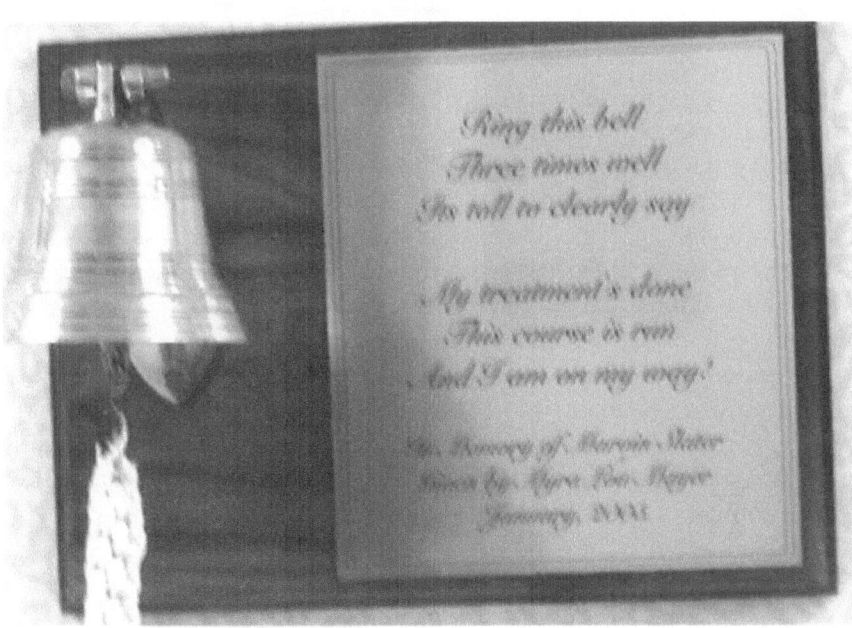

TIME FOR SURGERY

September 5, we met Paula's cousin Robin and his wife, Louise, at the airport. They flew to Houston from Iowa. This is the second time I have met them, and they came to be with me while she is in surgery and to help when we go to the apartment; this means so much to me. We have been fortunate enough to find this apartment through an organization known as "Open Arms" that helps medical patients with lodging when they come in from out of town. It is a real nice apartment complex. It is approximately twenty years old, but very well maintained. This will help defray the financial burden. It is thirty miles north of Houston, but such a clean and quiet complex. This evening, we drive to Kemah Boardwalk with Robin and Louise; they have never been to that place, and it was great. Paula and Louise rode several rides and laughed like little girls. We ate, and Robin and I sat and talked about their younger days. It has been about two years since Robin and Paula had visited each other.

September 8, we drove to Galveston. This day was perfect. The weather was great, cool enough to be comfortable, blue skies and lots of people walking around and having a good time. We stopped in several souvenir shops and went to eat. Watching Robin and Paula was great. To hear them tell stories of when her dad was alive and Robin going to visit for the summer when he was a kid, you could see her eyes light up. She was reliving those days through the stories. We then went to the Sixty-First Street, Fishing Pier, and sat at the top while watching people fishing, the wind blowing and oldies music played. After we left there, Paula and Louise walked barefoot on the beach. While they were walking, Paula had on flip-flops, and one of them broke, so we traveled to Murdoch's. Not just another souvenir shop, it is Paula's favorite. This one was built around 1903 and has survived many hurricanes. There are very large clamshells on the steps leading to the shop.

Open on both front and back so that the breeze blows through. We sat on the deck, overlooking the ocean, and relaxed. It was good that Robin and Louise were there for Paula.

September 9, Paula is in good spirits going in for the bilateral mastectomy. I can't help but worry. Robin sat in the waiting room and slept most of the day; he did not sleep too well at the apartment. Louise and I worked word-seek books and talked about Paula and her family to pass the time. The surgery took several hours, but when Dr. Lucci came out, he said everything looked really good. From what he saw, there was no sign of cancer in none of the lymph nodes, tissue, or skin. When I finally got to see her in recovery, she was so sleepy, but she was still as beautiful as ever. This night would be a long night as I would not leave her side; I slept in a chair in the room with her.

September 10, this morning, she is discharged, and we go to the apartment. Paula is doing well; we have both watched the video on how to maintain her drains. We have to go back at 5:00 p.m. for Herceptin maintenance. We get to the apartment and she goes into the bedroom and looks into the mirror. I thought this would be the time she would breakdown, but she stood there and just looked, turning from side to side, and looking at the bandage that was wrapped around her chest. She noticed that I was standing there and never said a word, no tears. But I felt she was crying inside because now she felt less of a woman. I feel so bad for her, but she is strong and will get through this.

Ike Is Coming

We are watching the weather on a local newscast, and there is a hurricane coming. Ike was his name. The reporters are saying how bad this hurricane is, and when it makes landfall, it will be as wide as Texas and travel all the way to Houston. We are not scheduled to leave until Thursday, September13, but Robin and Louise made plans to leave early, so we contacted the airline and changed our flight date to September 11.

Paula had reservations about flying on this date since September 11, 2001 was the terrorist attack in New York, but we found out when we got to the airport that they would be closing at 9:00 a.m. on Friday. There were so many people at the airport that it took a long time to get checked in and get through security. When we boarded the plane and were ready to depart, we had to wait on the runway for about thirty minutes because of all the planes leaving Houston Hobby. Paula slept most of the way to Nashville. The trip in the car to Bowling Green was painful for her. We also know that we have to be back in Houston on September 22 for a follow-up visit. That will be our wedding anniversary, so we have it planned to celebrate there. After we got home, I had no problem changing the dressing and emptying the drains that were attached to a belt that Paula had to wear. I would empty them before I went to work, come home at lunch, and then do it again before bedtime. Paula was so patient and understanding when I would move one of the drains and it would pull her skin, causing pain. This is one of the duties that a caregiver must contend with. I will say that I have had a lot of responsibilities through all of this, but I would not change one moment of it. Tempers can be short when you are in a situation like this, and I know that the kids are hurt sometimes because they will get too close to her, and I worry that one of them will do something to damage a tube or an incision. I am so tired, and they do pick up after themselves, but it bothers me that the oldest one will not help unless he is asked to.

As we get ready to head back, we get to the airport in Nashville, and I have her in a wheelchair going through the airport. When we start into the security area, Paula has to get out of the wheelchair and walk through the metal detector. The guard asked her to come through and stop, so she could use a handheld wand to scan her. Paula seemed to be a little embarrassed as she showed the guard the four hand-grenade-shaped plastic receptacles. There was another guard who saw them and noticed her wearing a cap with the pink ribbon on it. He commented on how his wife had been healed of cancer a few years before and wished her all the best and he would keep her in his prayers.

After the Hurricane

When we got to Houston, we immediately went to the emergency center as we had been instructed by her doctor. The emergency-center physician was not a nice person at all. She was ill tempered and not very friendly like most of the employees at MDACC. If you stop in a hallway or lobby and just look around, someone will ask you if you are lost or need help. We explained to her that we were there to have the drains removed because Dr. Lucci knew that two of the drain tubes were becoming infected, and he said when we got to the emergency center, they would remove them. But the doctor insisted that she be admitted. So here we are, all ready to celebrate our first anniversary in Houston, Texas, and we spend the night in the hospital. Paula is so depressed about this and kept apologizing to me, but I told her, "It's not where you're at, it's who you're with." And I was with the one I loved. I decided to go for something to eat and kept driving around, trying to find a restaurant that was open. I drove for over an hour, finally found a police officer, and asked him where the nearest place to get something to eat could be located. He told me that all of the restaurants were closed due to a curfew. I asked him why there was a curfew, and he explained about the severity of the hurricane in town and how every business was closing at 9:00 p.m. So I went back to the hospital room at around 12:00 p.m. so tired I could not stand up, and the nurses had Paula a food tray delivered to her room. This was the night from hell as all of our plans had been washed down the river. We will eventually get to have a first-year anniversary.

The next day, one of Dr. Lucci's fellows (a person who has completed almost all of their training) came into the room to examine Paula. She said that the drains should have come out the night before and then proceeded to remove them so we could get out and go to her scheduled appointments. When we got to the breast center, Dr. Lucci came in with his assistant, all smiles, and exclaimed that there is "NO CANCER AT ALL." The chemotherapy did its job, and she is cancer free at this time. He also told us that maybe one time a year, they get to give this kind of report to a patient where the patient responds this well to chemotherapy. I was so overjoyed that I could not speak. There is a 1 percent to 5 percent chance of it ever recurring, but it could come back. We met a geneticist named Pournema. She is a very nice lady who works in the genetics department. Paula has agreed to participate in a program that will format her family history and possibly tell the probability of her children ever getting cancer. There is a lot of paperwork to fill out.

September 25, Dr. Eleni came in to see Paula and asked her if she would talk to another patient. This woman named Marty and her husband came to Houston from Florida, so Paula and I talked to them, explained the process, and told them of her results. It turned out that she had cancer previously and came to MDACC, this time hoping for a cure. Tonight we went to eat; there was Marty and her husband at the same restaurant, so we sat and talked for a while. I often wonder how she is doing with her treatments.

LOCAL TREATMENTS OR NOT

Paula finally gets to drive since her mastectomy. Not the best drive to be making, but to the local medical center to fill out forms for starting radiation treatments and have records transferred from MDACC. The radiation specialist at our local cancer center is Dr. McGahan. He treated my mother of throat cancer and is very nice and caring, but Paula has some reservations about going here because she has been going to MDACC for all of her other treatments. If we go back to Houston, it will be radiation treatments two times a day for four weeks, or we could stay six weeks and only have one treatment a day.

Paula does not want to spend the extra two weeks away from her sons, so there is a big decision to make—stay home or go to Houston. We both met with a doctor at the medical center in Bowling Green and she was so rude and sarcastic. She acted like this particular type of cancer was nothing at all. I did not like her and had made up my mind that we should go to Houston. It turned out that she did not even work for the medical center but was standing in for Dr. McGahan while he was out of town. The technician who would be doing the treatments came in and talked with us for a while. She seemed knowledgeable, but did not convince me this was the best place for Paula. After all, Paula had promised to give me fifty years of marriage, and I was willing to do whatever it takes to see that fifty years.

Long Drive to Texas

Friday, October 17, was just like any other day at work. When I got home from work, Paula announced to me that she wanted to go to Houston for her radiation treatments. This was such short notice. I immediately called my partner and explained to him that we were going to Houston for her radiation treatments so he could handle the workload. He said he could and told us to have a good trip. I called my secretary and told her so she would know that I would not be back for a month. At 5:30 p.m., we left out for Texas with our two dogs. Driving until around midnight, we stopped in Palestine, Arkansas, checked into a small motel, and slept until the morning. We got up at six thirty, got started on the road again, and followed the directions I had printed from the computer map. For driving that far, which turned out to be approximately seven hundred miles, our two dogs did really well. We got to the apartment on Saturday afternoon and settled in so that Paula could lie down. She was tired, and I could see it in her eyes and hear it in her voice. We rested for a few hours and decided to get something to eat, so we went to a Mexican restaurant close to the apartment. Paula had a fruity drink, as this would be one of the last times she could have on for a while.

Sunday, October 19, around 11:00 a.m., I went back to the restaurant to get some salsa and chips. It has to be the best I have ever eaten; this will be my breakfast. We had to be at the Texas Medical Center for a blood draw and chest X-ray at 1:00 p.m. We went back to the apartment after the tests and lay around watching television. Later that evening, we took the dogs for a walk through a subdivision. The weather is so warm, and the walk is great for Paula's spirit and health. When we got back to the apartment, Paula fell asleep on the couch and stayed there for several hours before going to bed. She slept well for a change. Every day seems to make her a little weaker, but she keeps going and never complains about any pain.

Monday, October 20, 2008, starts off with a CT scan. After that, we went to the infusion therapy so they could put this long large needle in her port. I don't really know why this was done, but it really hurt her, and she cried. It about breaks my heart when something hurts her so bad she cries. She finally went for the CT scan, which took a long time. When she was finished with that, we went to eat because we were starved, some days you do not get to eat on a regular basis. Sometimes, the days are very long, getting paperwork completed, tests, prescriptions, and appointments. Tomorrow, she will receive the first of many radiation treatments. There have been many times we did not leave the clinic until 9:00 pm, and then it was a thirty-five-minute to one-hour drive to the apartment.

Tuesday, October 21, we're at the clinic early for preparation to start radiation therapy. It only took one hour to have the procedure completed. As Paula was in the treatment room, I worked on a jigsaw puzzle to occupy my time. There are puzzles and other items placed around the room for family or friends to work on.

RADIATION BEGINS

When she came out, she had multiple lines drawn on her chest and lower portion of her neck. I remarked that she looked like a road map; there were red, blue, and orange, and violet horizontal and vertical lines. Each line represented the different amounts and angles of radiation. We met with Dr. Wendy Woodward to check the placement of the lines, and she could answer any questions.

October 22 starts out with a trip to the library to use a computer to book a flight for Brad and Logan to come to be with us because Paula did not want to be away from them so long. After the library, we went to the Woodlands Mall for her to take some pictures. She got out of the car to photograph a building. She was walking down the street and slipped in some water where she fell and bruised her knee. It seems every time we come to Texas, she falls and hurts herself. Once again, it's time to go back to the clinic for a "dry run simulation" that starts at 4:30 p.m. and does not end until 7:30 p.m . . . By now it has started to rain, and lots of it. This is one of the hardest rains I have ever seen, and we have to drive back to the Woodlands in it. It took all of one and a half hour to go thirty miles. We talked about the starting of the real radiation treatment tomorrow and how it would affect her. I am worried how bad she will burn and her energy level.

Thursday, October 23, starts at 4:00 a.m. as we have to be at the clinic at 6:30 a.m. and I oversleep. We rushed around to get ready and did not get to eat, but the drive in was good and went reasonably quick. She checked in, went back, and had completed the treatment within thirty minutes. I thought this is not going to be as bad I had imagined. We drove back to the apartment to let the dogs out and spend the day resting until time to go back in the afternoon. We rest a lot because the chemotherapy still has not completely left her body.

Each day will be two trips into town for around thirty minutes. If we did not have the dogs, we could spend the day in Houston or surrounding area, but we have to go let them out. The treatments will eventually make her more tired and start to burn her skin. When she started the first day of treatments, we were given a schedule of appointment times; so at the end of each treatment, I draw a black line through it. It doesn't seem as though forty treatments is that many, but when you look at it on paper, it can be overwhelming. At least there will be no treatments on the weekends.

Sunday, October 26, we decided we would go to Lakewood Church in Houston. Joel and Victoria Osteen broadcast from there, which we had watched on television in Bowling Green. When we arrived, the ushers sat us in the third row. All visitors for the first time sit in the front three rows. The sermon was about extraordinary people. I found this a remarkable service as Pastor Osteen spoke of God not letting ordinary people have extraordinary challenges. It seemed as though God had spoke to him about Paula. So this church, which used to be a basketball arena, seats eighteen thousand people. It is so overwhelming to be in a building with that many people worshiping at the same time. During a special prayer, Paula was led to the front by an usher, where she was prayed for by Mr. Osteen's mother, Dodie. She seemed to know that Paula and I had made plans for fifty years of marriage without being told. We tried to get to meet Mr. and Mrs. Osteen, but were unsuccessful this trip. We have decided that when we come to Houston, this will be our church.

Another First

Monday, October 27, we decided to use the HOV (high-occupancy vehicles) lane to get to Houston. This lane is to be for autos with two or more passengers and is supposed to be faster, but it is still slow. We got downtown and got misplaced, as I like to call it. Paula said we were lost, but I knew we were in Houston; we had a good laugh about that. Each day brings something new to challenge my nerves driving in this enormous town.

We arrive, and she goes in while I park. I wait for her to call and come back to pick her up half an hour later. October 28, here we are, "LATE AGAIN." It seems that we can never be on time for the morning appointment. Paula is definitely not a morning person. The traffic is so bad coming in; we need to leave earlier, but she doesn't want to get up earlier so we can be on time. There is a sore that is on her right leg that is getting worse, and I am starting to feel bad. Today, we hope to see a dermatologist about the places that show up on her body. They get large and look as if they are infected. We don't know what it is. Dr. Woodward's nurse Shirley told us that she had gotten an appointment with a dermatologist scheduled for tomorrow.

October 29, we go to radiation, then dermatology. We saw a doctor, and they took a punch and removed a piece of tissue on her leg to send it to pathology for testing to see what type of infection it is. The Dr. thinks it is staph infection, which could have been the result of the surgery. This will take approximately three days for the results to come back. Until then she will have to take an antibiotic to help her get over the infection. With all of the procedures, chemotherapy, and radiation, she is subject to infections because she is so weak. Chemotherapy has weakened her immune system, which is common with cancer patients. We struggled through the day as both of us felt bad. I think I have some type of infection myself, or maybe I am just tired from the two trips a day. The next day is nothing but treatments and back to the apartment. No additional plans for the day.

October 31, we were planning to go to the clinic and stay in town, so we took our dogs with us. During her radiation treatment, she started feeling real bad, so the doctor had her taken to the emergency center. So I had to drive back to the apartment with the dogs, and then drive back to the hospital where she was. We were there until 3:00 p.m., but the doctors did not do anything. Her afternoon treatment was at 4:00, so we got back to the apartment around 6:30 p.m. This has been the most difficult day since we have been here. I am starting to feel worse as time goes by.

November 1, 2008, brings a new day. We are getting ready to go to the airport and pickup Brad and Logan this afternoon. I woke up this morning and felt so bad. My whole body hurts, and I have no energy whatsoever. We were told of a shorter way to the airport they were flying into, but I was not sure of this route, so I went the long way. That was a mistake. There was an accident, which had traffic to a complete stop, and Paula was getting upset that we would not get to the airport on time when they got off the plane. This is the first time they have flown by themselves, so Paula was scared to death. Cathy and Donnie put them on the plane in Nashville, and we were to receive them in Houston.

We drove to the wrong place at the airport, which had her more upset, but the security guard told us to leave the car where we had parked, and he walked us to the terminal where they would be. She was so glad when she saw them that her energy level seemed to go straight to overdrive. Mine was still in low gear. While they are with us, she is going to home school them, which I thought was a bad idea as she would not feel like it, because I was afraid they would get behind in their studies. While they are with us, we do some fun things and they are having a good time.

November 2, 2008, and my symptoms are getting worse. Thank God it is Saturday. Paula felt a little better today, so she went to the grocery, bought food, and purchased me mixed fruit and watermelon chunks. I ate the mixed fruit and laid back down, feeling worse than ever. This was the longest day I believe I have ever seen. I feel so bad, and I am not able to take care of Paula as I am supposed to.

November 3, 2008, we go for her regular round of treatments. She is feeling better, but I still feel terrible. After radiation, we go to the dermatologist, and she wrote me a prescription for the same infection that Paula has. I need to get better so I can help Paula.

CHANGES

November 4, 2008, is a better day for me, I don't feel as bad as I have the past few days, but still pretty lousy. Her redness is getting worse, and the pain is beginning to increase. I have started to put a cream and a type of petroleum jelly on her chest to help ease the pain and redness. Also, I have to put antibiotic ointment on her leg and bandage it from the punch biopsy. She is so tender to the touch, and the heat radiating from her chest melts the petroleum jelly so it slides off pretty quickly. Paula is tolerating the radiation well, but I know that she is hurting even though she does not complain about it. There have been times that she can barely put on her nightshirt or blouse without grabbing it in front and holding it from touching her skin. I feel so bad that there is nothing I can do to help her, except apply the cream and ointment.

Every day that passes gets worse for me and Paula. I am so tired; this infection is getting me down, but I have to keep going to help her. It has gotten to the point that I feel helpless and useless to her. Paula is getting so tired and sluggish now. Only sixteen treatments out of forty, and she is this tired and burned. I don't know if she will be able to take this, and if that is not enough, she has physical therapy at 4:00 p.m. to stretch the muscles and tendons in her arms from her bilateral mastectomy. While we were in the waiting room, Paula met Gertrude, a lady from Pakistan who was there with her husband, Dennis. He had been through chemo and was now doing his radiation. She told us of how she had been a preschool teacher and her husband being transferred to Houston with the company he worked for. She had been diagnosed, treated, and cancer free for sometime now. It really is amazing how many people you can meet and hear interesting stories of their past history of cancer and of being healed. She sat and talked with me while Paula was in for her treatments. Then there was "Ms. Annie," a little sweet lady that came from Beaumont, Texas. She has no family and rode a bus that brought her. Paula just fell in love with her. Sometimes we talk about "Ms. Annie." I keep telling Paula that she needs to call and see how she is doing. "Ms. Yvette" was an employee who was so gracious with Paula's boys, and on the last day of treatments, she brought them a present as a reminder of her. Each day is exactly the same as the day before, treatments and back to the apartment. With every treatment, the burning gets worse and the pain more intense. I had talked to my older brother Bruce in South Carolina about another brother Melvin in Tennessee who was diagnosed with pancreatic cancer and had been through all of the treatments about the same time that Paula was diagnosed. Melvin had not tolerated the radiation well. Bruce told me on the phone that Melvin had burned so bad that he was giving up and looked like a piece of burned bacon. I feel so guilty because I did not get to go visit Melvin before he passed away.

THE END OF RADIATION

Nineteen more treatments and we get to go home for a while. November 19 and Paula finishes her radiation treatments. She gets to "RING THE BELL" today. The customary ringing of the bell signifies that you have completed another milestone in your journey through cancer. After each treatment, Paula walks by this bell and reaches out, touches it, and dreams about the day she will ring it. You also get to ring the bell when you finish chemotherapy, but Paula was in Bowling Green for her last chemo treatment, so she did not get to ring the bell in Houston. It was a glorious day when she walked up to the bell, caressed it, and made her speech that how she appreciated everything that the technicians had done for her. All the while, I was videotaping this occasion while Bradley had Cathy on the phone listening as Paula rang the bell of freedom. Freedom of breast cancer and no more painful treatments. Paula had more energy at that moment than she had in weeks. Her smile and her fervor were insurmountable. She cried as I did, but no one knew that I was crying. I am so proud of the way she has come through all of this. I don't think there is any way I could have tolerated what she has been through the past forty days.

We will start our long journey home tomorrow, but tonight we will celebrate. On November 20, Cathy called to tell us of the weather at home because as we leave Texas, it is in the sixty-degree range. We drive as far as possible, only stopping to use the bathroom and let the dogs use the bathroom. Paula is doing well with the trip so far. We pulled into Timpton, Texas, to get gas, breakfast, and let the dogs walk around. I met a cute elderly gentleman Red Davis, who informed me in a funny tone to get the "hell out and never look back at this godforsaken town." He had been trying to sell his farm for thirty years, but not too hard. This is a small charming town; I think I could live here. Her burning is getting worse, but her spirit is good. She loves this one particular building that is very small with barn siding and looks like something out of an old West movie.

It houses a beauty shop. She took several pictures of it on the way to Houston, and now she is taking pictures of the same building. The trip is uneventful and very cold when we arrive.

November 25, we are finally at home, and Paula's chest is looking very bad now. Every time she moves, she cries out, just to lay down causes severe pain. She is in such pain; she woke me up at 2:30 a.m. and told me that there were fire trucks outside. There is a house down the street that caught fire from a car fire. I tried to go back to sleep but was unable, although she fell asleep quickly. I start getting the boys ready for school while she sleeps; she needs all of the rest she can get.

November 27 is Thanksgiving Day, and I have a lot to be thankful for. I have Paula with me. We met her family for Thanksgiving lunch, and her niece Marla took her for a ride in a Corvette. They were riding with the tops off of the car; she had a smile as big as I have ever seen because she was enjoying life. She still takes Herceptin maintenance and has to go tomorrow for that. I know that she does not feel like it, but she has to go.

Bad Day at Hospital

We get to the medical center for the Herceptin. The nurse puts Paula in a hospital room, starts an IV, and leaves to get the medicine. The nurse comes back and announces, "We do not have it and cannot get it." I was so upset that I called a hospital administrator and told them this would be a good place to start a hospital, to which I was informed that she would investigate and let me know the results of why they did not have and could not get the medication needed. This maintenance drug is crucial in the preventive part of cancer treatment. With the pain and blistering, Paula is hurting so bad, but should start to get better soon. This is not a bad hospital, but they do not specialize in cancer therapy like MD Anderson. I think this is the reason that we have bad experiences every time we go there.

THE INFECTION

Saturday, November 29, starts off different. Paula got out of bed, went straight to the recliner, and stayed there most of the day. She called Dr. Woodward's office in Houston and got the on-call doctor. She suggested that we go on to the emergency room and get checked out. Dr. Thomas, the emergency-room doctor, called the local oncologist that treats to get permission to admit her. After three calls to the oncologist and three times her saying no to admitting Paula, Dr. Thomas called Dr. Fentress, the hospitalist, who came in and admitted her. She got to the room and the nurses started an IV, and she started getting some relief. She had a multitude of doctors and nurses come during the night and the next morning.

Dr. Campbell, a surgeon, came in, looked at Paula's chest, and was going to take her to a surgery suite to remove the dead tissue so that the healing would begin all over again. Then Dr. McGahan came in and stated that the same procedure could be done in her room with the use of extra pain medication. A pain management nurse came in to start the procedure and was very gentle with her. Paula was in the hospital for approximately four days and released. It would be up to me to change the dressing, two to three times a day, and clean the affected area and redress her chest.

Removing the dressing and cleaning the infected area is not difficult, but when I remove the gauze pads, they seem to stick to the skin somewhat, and it causes tremendous pain. It hurts her, but she knows that I am being as gentle as I can. It hurts me emotionally to cause pain to Paula because I love her so much. The healing is coming along slowly, but looking better each day.

We have to be back in Houston on January 6 for a test to see if Paula will be well enough for the next surgery. This surgery will be to remove the tumor from her duodenum, a tube between the stomach and the intestine. We have to be at the clinic at 1:00 p.m. so they can start the preliminary procedure. We left Bowling Green at 5:00 p.m., Monday, January 5, and stayed at the Hotel Preston in Nashville. We had to be at the airport at 5:00 a.m., be checked through security, and board the plane at 6:00 a.m. I was apprehensive about getting on this plane as it was so small. It only seated fifty persons. We were so cramped that I bumped my head three times just getting seated. About one and a half hour into the flight, we encountered some serious turbulence and were bounced around very bad. My decision was definite; I will not fly back on one of these planes. Paula still has a lot of tenderness in her chest from the infection. The plane ride did not help her at all. To feel the clothing touch her skin was still painful.

We made it to the clinic Tuesday afternoon, and the technician gave Paula this liquid to drink. I took a small sip to see how it tasted, and it was bad. Paula had to drink four liters of this foul-tasting liquid over a three-hour period. She did not get much sleep that night as she was up and down going to the bathroom, but at least tomorrow she would sleep.

There were several people there getting prepared for the same test, and it took a long time for them to get ready for her. We did not leave the clinic until 9:00 p.m. and had to be back the next morning at 6:00 a.m., so Paula could not have anything to eat anything.

Wednesday morning, we arrived at the hospital at 6:00 a.m., got checked in, and were ready for the "colonoscopy." By now, Paula is tired and very hungry; and when we get finished with this, she has other appointments and tests. The procedure lasted fifteen minutes, and all went well. We met with an internal-medicine doctor, and she said everything is good, so the surgery will proceed as planned. Paula and I are going to Kemah, Texas, tomorrow to see how much they have rebuilt since the hurricane. During times of illness, a person really needs to get away and enjoy time out when there are no appointments or tests.

January 9 starts off good. We go to the clinic to see Dr. Abdalla for preoperative meeting. After visiting with him, he informs us that the surgery will be postponed for at least a week because she has problem with her voice. She does not have a cold but simply lost her voice. Dr. Abdalla was insistent that she wait because of the tube that would be placed in her throat could cause her to go into pneumonia. Now we have to wait until January 20. Sometimes I feel like the world is against me, Paula having cancer, then surgeries, and infections.

Now the waiting just makes it worse. We take trips to different places that are close to enjoy the time we have together before the surgery. We went to a very nice restaurant that was located in the Woodlands; we had a late dinner, and we tried mussels for the first time. With Paula, I have had so many first experiences. We enjoy this town so much I believe I could move there. The people are a little different, but for the most part, they are friendly.

FINAL SURGERY

It is finally time for surgery. And yet another delay. We get to the clinic only to find out that there has been an electrical failure in the surgery suite. While Paula was in the pre-op area, the nurse and the anesthesiologist came in to place an epidural pain block in her back. She was supposed to go in for surgery around 10:00 a.m. but did not get in until 1:00 p.m. The surgery was to last between four to six hours, so I was in the waiting room, working word puzzles and reading magazines. At 2:15 p.m., the surgery nurse came out to let me know how she was doing. Everything was going well. Around 3:00 p.m., I thought I would go downstairs to get me a soft drink and snack, so I informed the volunteer that I was leaving for a few minutes, when the nurse told me that the doctor wanted to speak with me, I was so terrified that something had happened. I started to imagine the worst things you could think of. The nurse was taking me to a small consultation room. When I saw the doctor coming down the hallway and asked him what was going on, he told me, "I have done all I can do." That sounded to me like it was worse than he thought. She was okay, so I asked him why the surgery only took two hours and fifteen minutes when it was supposed to be a four-to six-hour surgery, and he told me she was a textbook case. Everything went as planned. He also advised me that he had done a biopsy on her liver because there were some spots that did not look right, and he also removed her gallbladder at the same time. It turned out that the spots on her liver were nothing to be concerned with. I was so relieved and started making the phone calls to her family and friends that wanted to know when it was over.

Wednesday, January 21, turned out to be a little better day for Paula. She slept most of the day with the help of pain medication. The nursing assistant came in, got her up in a chair, and bathed her, which was hard since she had an NG (a.k.a. "nose hose") tube down her nose to remove the fluid from her stomach.

She was able to sit in a chair for about twenty minutes before having to get back in bed. In the late afternoon, we got her up and walked her around the nurse's station two times, and she was so tired and sore. I was so proud of her; she had stated before her surgery that she was going to try as hard as she could to get out of the hospital in four days. While I was going to a room around the corner from her room to get me a cup of coffee, I ran across this elderly gentleman who had just had the same surgery as Paula. He informed me that he had no pain at all, and when I told this to Paula, she stated with sarcasm, "Well, he is a man." To which I laughed. It turned out that he had had an epidural nerve block the same as Paula had. His worked and hers did not. That is why she was in pain, and he wasn't. Tonight, she slept very well, except when the nurse came in and woke her up to check her vital signs or take her temperature. I stayed in the chair beside her bed the whole time so that she would not be alone. I left only long enough to shower and change clothes.

On Thursday, January 22, the NG tube started to leak, so the nurse came and had to change her sheets on the bed and change her hospital gown. After all of that was done, we took a walk around the nurse's station again. This time, she was able to walk three times around it, which is fairly large, and it was a strain on her. But she completed the three trips. I sit in the chair, watch television, or do the word-puzzle books while she sleeps. Sometimes, I write in a notepad to keep account of the days and what happens. January 23, we were awakened at 4:30 a.m. when the nurse came in to take the vital signs. We were not able to go back to sleep, so we watched television and talked about the surgery and how well she was doing. At 7:30 a.m., the doctor came in and told us that she would be getting the catheter removed so she could move around a little more freely. Paula was more concerned with the tube in her nose, but it has to stay in for a few more days. We walk around the nurse's station three more times today. I want to do this several times a day, but she is just no able to yet. The oxygen level gets turned down, so maybe this means she will get rid of the oxygen tube today or tomorrow. Possibly, she will get the NG tube out tomorrow as well. What a relief, as I know this has to be painful. This is just one more step toward going home. Every day is a little bit better than the day before.

January 24 is here, and Paula is distraught that she is in a hospital, and today is Logan's birthday. She called him on the phone although she feels really bad today. The pain is not easing too much, it gets better then it comes back as bad as before. The doctors said it is normal for this to happen with this type of surgery. Not only has she been through a major surgery, but she also has not eaten anything since her surgery, and she is really weak. Even though she has not eaten, she is not saying too much about being hungry. Today, they gave her some ice chips to crunch on, and that seemed to make her hungry. Tomorrow I will try to help her get into the shower; maybe that will make her feel better, and we can walk around the nurse's station.

January 25, the doctor came in and said that she could have thirty cc's of liquid today. That sounds like such a little amount, but when you have not had anything for five days, it is a lot. She could only have that amount over a twenty-four-hour period, which turned out not to be the case. The doctor came back in and told her that she could have as much as she wanted to drink. The next day she was able to eat a solid meal, and eat she did. I think she ordered everything on the menu and ate every bite. After she ate and rested for a while, I got her in a wheelchair and took her on a short ride to the gift shop located in the clinic. There was a purse there that she fell in love with on a previous trip, and she wanted to see if it was still there. It was, and I purchased it for her while she was looking at some other items, and she was ecstatic. She wants to try to find a pair of matching shoes when she is released from the hospital, which we will go on a shopping spree, to find them when she is released. We have been here since January 20, and Paula is being discharged from the hospital eight days after she was admitted. We are going back to the apartment today and get settled in for another two weeks of rest for her. Before we leave, we explained to the doctor that she really needs to get the Herceptin maintenance treatment. He is doing what he can to get this set up as this is a cancer hospital, so it should not be an issue. While we wait for the Herceptin, Dr. Mason from pain management came in to see her and see how she was tolerating the pain. We finally get to leave and go back to the apartment, and it has turned cold. Paula talked to her sister, and Cathy told her that there was snow and ice at home, so we were glad to be in Texas.

We go back to the clinic on January 30 to see the doctor for a follow-up visit. Dr. Abdalla finally came in and told us of the type of tumor that he removed and explained that it was a GIST (gastrointestinal stromal tumor). He stated that if you had to have a tumor, this is the one to have, but he wanted her to see another specialist, Dr. Trent. We will have another trip back in a few weeks to visit him. Dr. Trent is definitely concerned with the tumor that was removed and let us know that there is a 10 percent chance that it could come back if preventive measures are not taken, so Paula started on an oral chemotherapy medication that is very costly. If it were not for insurance, she would not be able to get it. She has to take this medicine for one year. Paula has some of the side effects such as increase in appetite. We have been back in Bowling Green since January 30, and I am trying to help her with the daily chores still, until she gets better and pain free. Since the last surgery, she is continuing to get better, and the pain level from the surgery is decreasing, and soon Paula will be back to excellent health. The Herceptin will be over soon, and her medications are decreasing. She is only taking five medications daily, but every day is baby steps toward renewed health. Being a newly married couple and finding out that your spouse has breast cancer is frightening, not to mention finding out there are three different cancers in her body. It can be a strain mentally and physically, but you must have confidence in the physicians and everyone involved with the healing process.

It is now April of 2009, and Paula has returned to work full-time, and I am still doing the same as before, helping with the daily chores around the house as well as working full-time. Each day, she regains a little more strength and stamina. I am very confident that soon she will be back to her normal state of well-being.

The whole experience has been enlightening and very terrifying to a newly married couple, but I would not have changed one minute of one day for any thing in the world. I only hope and pray each day that I will get fifty years of love and companionship from this woman. Paula is much stronger than I would be, to endure all of the tests and surgeries.

Every day is full of new prayers from friends and acquaintances for Paula's health and well-being. We do not have to return to our second home of Texas until July 2009. **The one and only thing to remember is believe in God, and all illnesses can be healed.** I wear my pink rubber bracelet, and Paula still wears her pink ball cap sometimes. This is to let people know that we support cancer research, and have been touched by cancer. By doing this we both have met so many people who have a survivor story and they want to hear about her story.

WHODATHUNKIT!!!

April 27, 2009